Praise for *Primal Uprising*

"Read this book to learn what the founders of Paleo *f(x)* have learned about how to hack your health. Health isn't really about being healthy; it's about earning the freedom that comes from having the energy and the power to show up in your life. Lots of great advice here!"

—Dave Asprey, *New York Times* bestselling author of *The Bulletproof Diet*

"There are amazing lessons from our ancestors that can dramatically upgrade our model life. *Primal Uprising* merges ancestral principles of wellness with the technological advances of the modern world to facilitate deep, meaningful health. Michelle and Keith Norris are true crusaders who present an accessible, sustainable vision of health that encompasses every aspect of our lives from deep within us to far beyond us."

—J. J. Virgin, celebrity nutritionist, Fitness Hall of Famer, and *New York Times* bestselling author of four titles including *The Virgin Diet* and *The Sugar Impact Diet*

"The journey to optimal health is highly personal. Each individual will have different contributing factors, different goals, different genetics, and a different environment. Yet, there are some things that hold true for everyone, and in *Primal Uprising*, Michelle and Keith Norris have taken something very complex and confusing made it simple and clear with the seven pillars of health. What I love most about this book is that they focus less on rules and more on resilience. I believe resilience is the greatest path to health and something I spent the most time covering in my book as well. It's time to reframe 'stress' and this book shows you how to build that resilience with each pillar, which is brilliant. I read this cover to cover and it is something we all need right now."

—Shawn Wells, MPH, RD, LDN, CISSN, CISSN, bestselling author of *The Energy Formula*, biochemist, dietitian, and dubbed as "World's Greatest Formulator"

"As a metabolic scientist, my perspective on optimal health is viewed through the lens of the food we eat. However, while food matters, it alone fails to shine light on all facets of a sound body and mind. In *Primal Uprising: The Paleo f(x) Guide to Optimizing Your Health, Expanding Your Mind, and Reclaiming Your Freedom*, Michelle and Keith Norris illuminate seven diverse and distinct dimensions of human health and wellness that create a comprehensive view and strategy to a long and productive life."

—Benjamin T. Bikman, PhD, author of *Why We Get Sick* and associate professor of physiology and developmental biology at Brigham Young University

"Leverage the wisdom in this transformative book to enhance the human system and upgrade your life experience into a life of excellence!"

—Dr. Mickra Hamilton, cofounder and CEO of Apeiron

"Some of us like to live on the edge, experimenting with our health using all the resources available to us, but genuine full-spectrum health isn't just biohacks and better diets. Health is about looking at your whole life and changing the parts that aren't working. That's what Michelle and Keith have done in *Primal Uprising*, a stupendously comprehensive approach to health that covers food and movement, mind and emotion, spirit and human connection, money and tribe. It's about changing yourself to change a world in need of an evolutionary kick in the ass. As someone who obsessively considers every aspect of health, and who has recently focused on the less obvious aspects of human optimization like spirituality, family, and becoming a better person, I appreciate what they've done and recommend this book to anyone who wants to take their health to the next level."

—Ben Greenfield, *New York Time* bestselling author of *Boundless* and *Fit Soul*, and the founder of Ben Greenfield Fitness and Kion

"We are in a world where science, technology, and closed belief systems have led us, with all our *smarts*, to the edges of extinction, but if we were *wise*, we would be integrating the deep truths of ancestral wisdom lineages with the advanced technology and science today and the proof of our 'smarts' would be harmony, sustainability, and a better future for our children and nature itself. *Primal Uprising: The Paleo f(x) Guide to Optimizing Your Health, Expanding Your Mind, and Reclaiming Your Freedom*, offers you real wisdom, the application of which will create sustainability, foster responsible use of technology, and more importantly, guide you to finding and using the most advanced technology of all, which lives and breathes within you."

—Paul Chek, holistic health practitioner and founder of Chek Institute

"Michelle and Keith Norris, founders of Paleo f(x), have created not just a conference but a full-on movement, bringing together thousands of people who want to explore how to live a modern lifestyle rooted in ancestral principles. You can see how ahead of the trends they are, just by seeing who presents at their conference. With their book, *Primal Uprising*, they are helping people find health freedom—freedom from fad diets and dogma—by simplifying health into a fantastic framework that anyone can relate to. I especially love their perspectives on financial, spiritual, and tribal resilience because these are so often overlooked when people think about health. Really, if you can't afford to be healthy, that's a problem, and if you can't find meaning or purpose, what's the point of health, and if you have no one to share your life with, it's a lonely path. It's just so important to go beyond the surface when it comes to truly understanding what health is about and Michelle and Keith have done just that, and beautifully."

—Molly Maloof, MD, adjunct professor in the Wellness Department of the School of Medicine at Stanford, healthspan-focused concierge doctor, biohacker, and futurist

PRIMAL UPRISING

PRIMAL UPRISING

The Paleo *f(x)* Guide *to* Optimizing
Your Health, Expanding Your Mind,
and Reclaiming Your Freedom

Michelle Norris, CEO, Founder, and Owner of **PALEO** *f(x)*™
and Keith Norris, CDO and Founder of **PALEO** *f(x)*™
with Eve Adamson

Challenge Authority, Defy Dogma, Demand Different

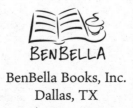

BenBella Books, Inc.
Dallas, TX

BenBella Books, Inc.
10440 N. Central Expressway
Suite 800
Dallas, TX 75231
www.benbellabooks.com
Send feedback to feedback@benbellabooks.com

BenBella is a federally registered trademark.

Printed in the United States of America
10 9 8 7 6 5 4 3 2 1

Library of Congress Control Number: 2020051903
ISBN 978-1-950665-85-3 (trade cloth)
ISBN 978-1-953295-25-5 (ebook)

Editing by Claire Schulz
Copyediting by Karen Wise
Proofreading by Kim Broderick and Greg Teague
Indexing by Guided by Words Indexing Services
Text design and composition by PerfecType, Nashville, TN
Cover design by Oceana Garceau
Cover illustration © iStock / Veida (hunter), taichi_k (smiley face), FreeSoulProduction (figures holding hands), kondratya (lotus blossom), str33tcat (infinity symbol)
Paleo FX logo courtesy of Dana M Norris, Paleo FX LLC
Printed by Lake Book Manufacturing

Special discounts for bulk sales are available. Please contact bulkorders@benbellabooks.com.

To Brittani.
Thank you for teaching us how to find beauty in the ashes, and inspiring us to continue your legacy of changing people's lives.

A prayer for the wild at heart kept in cages.

—TENNESSEE WILLIAMS

Contents

Are You Captive or Are You Free?

It had never occurred to him that an animal could be stripped of everything that went with it, of which its instincts were an inseparable part, and that you could have just its little body in a space of nothingness. As if looking at *that* told you anything but the nature of sorrow, which you knew anyway.

—Lucy Maria Boston, novelist

Have you ever noticed how animals behave in captivity? They don't act, or look, like their wild counterparts. Inside their cages, tanks, or enclosures, they pace, run in circles, self-harm, fight with each other, become destructive, have sudden bouts of madness. Eventually, their instincts become dull. They stop trying to hunt or forage because their food is dumped in front of them. They eat more than they need. They may stop playing, or even breeding. They become complacent, docile, out of shape, overweight. They give up and give in to a life in captivity.

Sound familiar?

Even when the enclosures are large or attempt to mimic the animal's natural environment, the animals are still in cages. The animals are still in a zoo. Are they safer? Perhaps. Life in the wild can be treacherous. Yet, a wild and free life can also be joyous. It is a life of self-reliance, requiring strength, speed, creative thinking, instinct. It is a life fully lived.

Which would you rather have? Safe, joyless captivity? Or dangerous, ecstatic freedom?

In many ways, our modern world is a human zoo, and you and everyone you know are the captives. It is a zoo of our own making. We have been led into our cages willingly, if not knowingly. We have been convinced, by institutions more powerful than any individual, that we require caretaking. That we can't think for ourselves. That we want to buy what they are selling, watch what they put in front of us, eat what they make easily available to us, and perhaps worst of all, believe what they tell us.

They tell us not to worry. Why worry over food when we have the drive-thru? Can't sleep? Take an Ambien. Can't relax? Here's a Xanax. Then there's Ritalin and Red Bull to see you through those all-nighters because hey, you've got to land and then keep that big corporate gig, right? The one that keeps you chained to a life you aren't sure you really want? But it's fine. You have nice things. Or, you want nice things. And the great part is, you don't have to fight to survive because it's all taken care of for you. Don't you fret. They've got this.

Or do they?

The truth is, while telling you not to worry, they keep you in fear so they can keep you under control. But it is not your destiny to be in a zoo. It is your destiny to have optimized health; a free and creative mind; generous productive emotions like love, empathy, and compassion; an understanding that you are a part of something much bigger than yourself; resources to fulfill your purpose; connection to other humans; and a deep, abiding sense of belonging. It is your destiny to live fully and freely in pursuit of happiness and meaning.

If that's what you want, then you are one of us, and if that's what we all want, then we are going to have to rise up and take our lives back. To do this, we will have to get stronger, smarter, and more emotionally intelligent. To escape the human zoo and claim our freedom, we will need to see beyond the narrow boundaries of our individual lives and ascend into a unified, resourceful, creative tribe that achieves health in mind, body, and spirit.

We believe true health can be achieved only by mastering each of the seven pillars of health: the physical, mental, emotional, spiritual, financial, relational, and tribal pillars that contribute to making a truly whole human. There are things you can do right now to begin living in accordance with your biological destiny and stepping into your full potential.

We're Michelle and Keith Norris, the cofounders of Paleo f(x), one of the premier holistic wellness conferences in the world, and the largest dedicated ancestral health conference in the nation. Our conference started as a deep dive into the diet of early humans and an exploration of how we might get back to those natural human roots, but with each passing year, "paleo" becomes something broader and bigger. We're not just the event anymore. We're the biggest repository of paleo-related information in the world. We're a platform, a movement. We are an uprising. It's the most exciting thing we've ever done.

But we didn't create Paleo f(x) randomly, and we didn't go down the rabbit hole of human optimization just for fun. We did it to feel better physically, and to become better humans. But most of all, we did it for Brittani.

Our Paleo Story

We met in high school. It was 1981. Keith was a junior, and a star football player. Michelle was a sophomore, and on the drill team. We hung with the same crowd, and we were both secretly in love with each other, but we were young and stupid and didn't want to ruin our friendship. We didn't yet recognize that friendship is the basis of a truly great relationship.

After high school, we stayed in touch. Keith got injured and had to end his career as an athlete, so he joined the military. Michelle had a string of different jobs, as she tried to figure out what she wanted to do with her life. We both got married to other people, but in 1999, we reconnected online while Michelle was searching for classmates to invite to our high school reunion, at a time when both our marriages were ending. Fast-forward to 2003, and we were married. It took us over twenty years to find our way back to each other, but once we did, we knew it was forever.

The idea of "paleo" wasn't on our radar in those days. We both had busy corporate careers and spent our time pursuing "the American Dream." We were happy together, if stressed by an intensely busy lifestyle, but one hitch in our happiness was Michelle's serious health symptoms. Every time she ate anything, she felt sick, but the doctors didn't seem to know exactly what was wrong. She was diagnosed with multiple chronic diseases, none of which seemed quite right: fibromyalgia, IBS, chronic fatigue syndrome, and early-onset rheumatoid arthritis. We couldn't understand it. We lived healthy lives. Michelle is a trained chef and her specialty was Italian cuisine. She cooked dinner at home every night with fresh whole ingredients. We hardly ever ate processed food or went out to eat. All that home-cooked food had to be good for us, or so we thought, yet Michelle's health continued to get worse.

Although Keith worked as a validation specialist for the pharmaceutical industry, he remained interested in athletic performance. To keep one foot in that world, Keith worked with a wrestling coach in North Carolina, helping the wrestlers maintain fitness between seasons so they could come back and "make weight." Keith knew that the rapid gains and losses wrestlers often enforce upon themselves are hard on the body, and he felt that this yo-yo effect was likely inhibiting performance. He suspected that performance would improve if the wrestlers could keep their weight more constant.

Specifically, he was thinking about manipulating body weight by altering carbohydrate intake. This has been a concept in the athletic realm since the 1950s, but Keith knew that the coach would want more than anecdotal evidence before advising his wrestlers to change their diets. Wrestling is a very traditional sport (like cycling and baseball), and to change anything about how it's done practically takes an act of Congress. Keith went in search of science in support of the relationship between carb intake and weight gain or loss as it applied to athletic performance.

Back in those days, when chat rooms were still a thing (this was around 2004 or 2005), Keith found one in which Robb Wolf and Art De Vany were members. This was before those guys were the renowned authors and speakers they are today. They were posting a lot about ancestral health and this "paleo" concept Keith had never heard of before. They kept mentioning gluten (the protein in wheat, rye, barley, and spelt) and saying it wasn't a part of the natural human diet. At the time, celiac disease was considered a rare condition. Most people hadn't heard of it, and "gluten-free" wasn't something in the mainstream consciousness.

Keith was intrigued, although he also thought it all sounded a little wacky (and told Robb and Art as much). Robb and Art began to send him scientific studies. These were mostly focused on health benefits of dietary changes, and Keith was more interested in performance, but then he thought about Michelle. Many of the articles about this so-called paleo diet described improvements in people with many of the same symptoms Michelle had. Maybe, Keith thought, this diet could help her. And, if these health benefits were so powerful, they might translate into performance benefits for the wrestlers after all. But to know for sure, he wanted first-hand experience, so he decided to try this weird new diet (which, as he later learned, was neither weird nor new) on himself.

At first, Keith didn't think the diet was having any effect on him. He had always been healthy and active, and he didn't feel any different . . . until the high blood pressure he thought was genetic suddenly normalized. That was a surprise. As he stuck with the diet, he began to realize subtle improvements. He had more energy, and his brain fog and constant need to eat resolved. His thinking was quicker and sharper. His performance improved in just about everything he was doing. And he became more and more convinced that this was a lifestyle that could help Michelle.

To Michelle, Keith's dietary changes seemed drastic. He was basically grain-free—something inconceivable to someone who specialized in making homemade pizza and pasta! Keith suggested Michelle try going gluten-free for thirty days as an experiment. What could it hurt? But Michelle couldn't imagine living without her favorite foods.

On the first day of his experiment, Keith made his own dinner. Michelle didn't think it could last, but he did it again the next day, and the next, and every time we sat down together, he suggested: "Maybe you should try this?"

"Nope. You and your crazy online friends can do what you want, and I'm going to eat what I want."

Keith stuck with it. What was originally just an experiment had become a lifestyle for him. One evening, about a year after Keith had "gone paleo," Michelle was making her kids' favorite homemade pizza for one of their birthdays, and she turned to Keith. "Are you really never going to have pizza or pasta again?"

"No, I'm not," he said. Then, for good measure, he added (again), "And you should get tested for celiac disease."

At last, impressed by Keith's commitment and obvious glowing health, Michelle relented and went to the doctor for a celiac disease test. Her results came back negative, but this was back when the tests weren't as accurate as they are now (they're still not infallible). Despite the test results, the doctor said he thought, based on her symptoms, that Michelle had some form of gluten sensitivity, and suggested she get a biopsy of her small intestine, which could confirm or rule out celiac disease definitively.

A biopsy? It sounded drastic and would require anesthesia. It didn't make sense to Michelle to do an invasive procedure *before* doing something as simple as changing her diet—something her doctor never mentioned. Maybe Keith was right. Why not try that first? Surgery-before-lifestyle seemed backward to Michelle, so she told the doctor no thanks (actually she said "Hell, no!"). She decided to try Keith's strange, counterintuitive diet, just to see if it helped. If it did, she would have her answer, no biopsy necessary. If it didn't, she could go back to her beloved carbs and look elsewhere. It was only thirty days.

Three weeks later, Michelle was still in a pretty big state of denial. She felt the inner conflict of desiring health versus desiring food, but then she noticed something surprising: Nearly all her symptoms had disappeared. It wasn't just not getting sick after eating anymore. The fatigue and pain were gone, including the chronic back and knee pain she'd thought were from rheumatoid arthritis. She was so used to living with the pain that she had accepted it as normal. Now that it was gone, she couldn't believe how good it felt to be without it. Maybe she didn't have rheumatoid arthritis, or the other problems, either.

Six weeks into her paleo experiment, everything changed. Michelle went to our son's first baseball game of the season, and everyone she knew who saw her noticed something different. They said things like:

"You look amazing!"

"How did you lose so much weight?"

"Why do you look so healthy?"

"Your skin is glowing . . . what have you done?"

All her friends were very familiar with "Michelle-on-a-diet." Dieting made her miserable. Her kids knew she would be in a bad mood if she was limiting her food intake. But this was something completely different. Michelle hadn't done any of that—she hadn't policed her portion sizes or counted calories, or done anything other than eat real whole foods without refined carbohydrates. Despite her initial resentment at not being able to eat those traditional Italian foods she loved, she had to admit that it had taken very little effort to change her food focus.

Keith likes to tell people that this was the day a paleo evangelist was born—because once Michelle is on board with something, everybody and their mother will know about it. If she thinks something will help people, she will shout it from the rooftops!

As time went on, these health realizations began to make Keith's Big Pharma job feel problematic. If people like Michelle could turn around serious health issues with diet alone, what was he doing putting all his energy and time into working for an industry that pushed drugs? There was a cognitive dissonance he couldn't reconcile.

Meanwhile, Michelle was working in property management, event planning, catering, then went on to study and work in architecture, technology, and construction management—she felt like she could do anything and everything, propelled by her newfound energy. At the same time, like Keith, she wondered if the industries she worked in were making a positive difference in the world.

Why optimize ourselves if we are going to use that energy and clarity only to keep financing our big house, our fancy cars, tuition at all the "best" schools, and more possessions than anyone needs? We began to feel handcuffed by the American Dream. We had to keep earning to keep up, and it felt like a trap. The healthier we got, the more we longed for an exit route. Funny how health can help you see more clearly. But we couldn't quite see how we could escape the grind.

Then the housing crisis hit in 2008, and our money evaporated in a big "fuck you" to our years of labor and perseverance. We couldn't believe everything we had worked so hard to acquire and maintain was gone. We began to wake up to the reality of our country's financial system, and the injustice of it all.

Then Brittani was killed.

We have a blended family of four beautiful children—Brittani, Kaley, Kleat, and Chase. Brittani was the oldest. She was intelligent, passionate, soulful, and excited to work in the mission field. At the age of twenty-two, she had already traveled all over the world helping others through her musical and spiritual gifts. Three days before her twenty-third birthday and one week before her college graduation, Brittani was killed in a car accident.

The next few months were a haze of pain and grief for us all. The two of us wondered what we were doing with our lives. We were spinning, unmoored. During her short dance on this earth, Brittani had already changed lives . . . so many lives. We held her first memorial service on what would have been her birthday, and nearly seven hundred people showed up. We stood in the receiving line for hours listening to people telling us how Brittani had helped them or made their lives better, in very specific and profound ways.

Soon after, we found out that there had been three memorial services for her in the US, one in South Africa, and one in Ireland. It was awe-inspiring. If someone so young could make such an impact, why weren't we changing the world for the better, too? We knew we had to carry on her legacy somehow. We asked ourselves, "What are our gifts?" We knew our passions: food, nutrition, health, fitness, and wellness. What could we do with that?

Our first idea was to create a foundation in Brittani's name with some kind of health and wellness theme, but we weren't quite sure how we would do it. Then in August 2011, we attended the inaugural Ancestral Health Symposium (a scientific conference that focuses on the science behind the paleo diet and lifestyle—see PrimalUprising.com/BookResources for more information). After the event, we were sitting on the runway at LAX. Michelle said, "That was a true symposium. Very academic. But wouldn't it have been cool to have some cooking demonstrations and more hands-on information about what people can actually do?"

Keith agreed. "It's an academic conference, not a lifestyle conference. They're not set up for that."

And then it dawned on us.

The notion that the way our ancestors once lived might contain wisdom and clues to optimal human health already fascinated us, but the missing component was a broad-scale, mainstream, interactive gathering that anyone could attend, understand, and benefit from. We envisioned bringing together experts who could explain how to use ancestral practices to improve modern life. We decided, right there on the runway, that we would create that event.

Our friends and family thought we had lost our minds. They warned us not to do it, but we had a vision and we had a calling. We knew we had to change our lives in a big way if we were ever going to make a big difference. On our anniversary a few months later, March 14, 2012, we launched Paleo f(x), and we had almost seven hundred attendees.

Paleo f(x) allowed us to transition out of work that was successful on paper but not in our souls to work that filled our souls but wasn't always successful on paper. We had some very difficult years. The "Bank of Norris" was financing Paleo f(x), and there were many times when we had enough to live on for two more weeks, or one more month. Yet somehow, the money always came through at the last minute. Each year, attendance grew a little more. Paleo f(x) became our primary occupation, and in 2019, we had a total of over 8,500 people attending the three-day conference. It's continued to grow since then.

Primal Uprising: The Future of Paleo

Today, Paleo f(x) has become a movement driven by many great minds, genius ideas, and the considerable energy that comes from those who live this lifestyle. For us, as for many, paleo started with diet, but it got bigger because of love and commitment, passion and purpose, and the urgency that comes from the realization that we are in real trouble if we allow ourselves to continue existing in docile captivity.

This is at the heart of everything we do now. There are systems—big systems, entrenched systems—that use their powerful reach and means to keep people down, unhealthy, on medications, depressed, anxious, foggy, isolated, lonely, and financially dependent. We must rise up and free ourselves if we want to reclaim our ancestral birthright and evolve into a better future.

Everywhere we go, we see the evidence that people are turning to the paleo lifestyle because they know they can no longer trust traditional resources when it comes to health, and they can tell we've gone too far in the wrong direction as a society. You only need to look at the global coronavirus crisis, or any other crisis the powers that be leverage to their own benefit, to see how abundantly clear it is that the government isn't going to change things. Massive corporations aren't going to change things. Why would they? Those groups are sitting pretty. They make money when we're not healthy—when we buy processed food and rely on pharmaceuticals and stay glued to our phones, living in fear. They have us right where they want us, but if you look up and look around, you'll see you don't have to remain under anybody's thumb.

The general public may still see paleo, if it is even on their radar, as just a diet. It may be easy to lampoon a movement purportedly based on cavemen with spears who don't use technology. But what those people don't understand is that the paleo movement isn't about copying what cavemen did. It's about utilizing modern technology and scientific wisdom to enhance human potential in a way that is fully in step with our ancestral instincts and our biological destiny, so that we can free ourselves from the human zoo.

As you can probably tell by now, this isn't a diet book. It's not a fitness book. It's not a book about mental health, or emotional well-being, or money, or human connection, or community, but it encompasses all those concepts because every one of them is necessary if we want our freedom back. This is a book about making the most of your body, mind, spirit, money, relationships, tribe . . . making the most of your entire life. It's also about making an impact, a contribution, a change for the better, in yourself and beyond. It's about changing you and, by extension, changing the world and the course of our very future.

The paleo movement opens a window to a new way of seeing. Whether it's the snack you choose or the skills you learn, the knowledge you acquire just for yourself or the activism you embrace for the greater good, this movement can awaken you to your purpose. Our mission is to help change your perspective because when perspectives change, actions change, and when actions change, people change, and when people change, the world changes, and only when the world changes will we all be free.

That is why we're here, and we think Brittani would be proud of us.

Primal Uprising Resources

In each chapter, we've included expert guidance from cutting-edge health practitioners, scientists, coaches, authors, spiritual guides, and activists. We also share many of our favorite companies, products, podcasts, books, and online resources. We want you to know, right up front, that we would never tell you what you should eat, do, take, use, or think. That goes against our whole message! We want you to learn about your own health in all its aspects and make your own decisions about how to optimize your health and your life. However, people often ask us what we do, what we use, what we take, and for those who are interested, we've created a web page containing information about everyone mentioned in this book, where to find out more about their services, and how to find the products and services we recommend. We also offer you a special readers-only discount on Paleo f(x) tickets for the upcoming event. Find all this information at PrimalUprising.com /BookResources.

PART I
THE
HUMAN
ZOO

One by one, the supposed attributes that we had thought were unique to humans have been shown to be present in other species. Crows use tools. Elephants can recognize themselves in a mirror. Whales form social networks of the same size and complexity as we do. Penguins mourn their dead. Gibbons are monogamous. Bonobos are polyamorous. Ducks rape. Chimpanzees deploy slaves. Velvet spiders commit suicide. Dolphins have language. And the quicker we get over the Judeo-Christian notion that we are somehow qualitatively different from the rest of the biome, the quicker we will learn to live healthier lives for ourselves and for the planet.

—Dalton Conley, professor of
sociology at Princeton University

1

YOU IN THE ZOO

The conscious and intelligent manipulation of the organized habits and opinions of the masses is an important element in democratic society. Those who manipulate this unseen mechanism of society constitute an invisible government which is the true ruling power of our country.

—Edward Bernays, from his book *Propaganda*

Reality check: Are we living in a human zoo?

You may not think you are, but let's consider the human condition as we know it today, in the twenty-first century. We work under artificial light. We eat artificial food. Our discussions, arguments, purchases, opinions, even our thoughts are largely shaped by social media and news that has become increasingly untrustworthy. We are dependent on medication, junk food, and sugar. We are told what's "best" for us, encouraged to be suspicious of those who are different (the ones in the other cages), and lulled into complacency that somebody else is in charge. We have become easily manipulated, inattentive, and emotionally reactive. We are kept, we are cowed, and we are controlled.

This, from where we are sitting, sounds like life in a zoo. We are metaphorically caged—just tired enough, stressed enough, and afraid enough to do what they tell us. How did we get here? When did life become so painfully predictable, sedentary, artificial, and confined? When did we become captives to the structures and systems created by our own human ingenuity?

As a species, humans were born free. Life was hard for our ancestors, sure. They had to build shelters, find food, and rely on each other. They had to think on their feet, and when they were in actual danger, they had to use their wits and speed to survive. They had to be strong and flexible, with endurance and fortitude, but they lived on their own terms, subject only to the fluctuations of the natural world.

Is there hope for our species, or are we doomed to a downward spiral of de-evolution? We believe there is hope, but only if we wake up and understand where we are, what we face, and what we need to do to re-create our lives in a free world. We wrote this book to be the guide for that awakening—the playbook for the primal uprising—because we believe that every one of us can embrace the past to reclaim the future.

Will you join us? Will you take the red pill or the blue pill? Let's dip a toe into the morass and see what's down there. Let's see if we can convince you that there is a better way to live than how we are living right now.

The Unnatural Nature of the Human Zoo

Are you safe in your cell? Maybe . . . sort of . . . but is that the kind of life you want? What if the choice is not one of safety versus danger, but of fearful captivity versus jubilant, challenging, growth-enhancing, blissful freedom that allows you to become more fully yourself?

You have the keys to the cell door. You have everything you need inside you right now to be a free human. You only need to access it and condition it. There is a way to wrest back control of your own life, food, environment, thoughts, emotions, beliefs, money, relationships, and tribe. You can question what you are told to think, and you can relearn how to think for yourself.

A friend once shared with us the way captive elephants are trained. When they are very young, a bracelet is put on their leg, and the bracelet is chained to a stake in the ground. The stake is stronger than a baby elephant, so when the elephant tries to walk away, it can't. It can move only as far away from the stake as the chain allows. The baby learns how far it can roam, and what its boundaries are. As the elephant grows, it quickly becomes large, strong, and fully capable of pulling that stake right out of the ground and running away. But it doesn't. It still believes it is limited by the boundaries its captors set for it from the beginning of its life. It stays chained, even though there is no reason why it can't set itself free.

This is called learned helplessness. The elephant believes that it can't escape, and so it never does, and that is the attitude of a captive. But it's not true that just because you have failed in the past, you will always fail, or that because you were told there are boundaries, or even shown actual boundaries, that there are still boundaries. If you believe, *I can't ever be that healthy, I can't ever be that strong, I can't ever be that happy, I can't ever feel good, I'll never have enough money, I can't find true love, I can't have real friends who accept me for who I am*, then you are self-limiting, like that elephant on the chain. An attitude of "I can't" is an attitude of scarcity, want, and powerlessness. Every limit that you think holds you back is just a story somebody told you about what you can or can't do. Do you believe the story?

What if you didn't? What if you knew you could pull out the stake and be everything you dream of? What if you didn't believe in those boundaries anymore? What if you had an attitude of "I can," of claiming your right to abundance, hope, creativity, and personal power? You can start wherever you are, recognize where you've been, and move forward into a more-empowered life.

If you choose to live in the human zoo because it is easier and more familiar, that is your right. You can sit back and wait for something bad to happen to you, then blame somebody else when it does. It's practically effortless to point a finger, or ridicule and get angry and troll the people who are doing or thinking something different from you. But ask yourself this: Would you rather be a spectator, or the one out there on the field, playing the game? If you would rather discover what's really true, and feel to your core how the zoo life you know is just an approximation of what real living is, then get ready.

The truth is that there is no stake in the ground. There is no cell door and there are no limits to what you can be. Human ingenuity is an eternal spring, and the power structures seeking to control you know that. That's what *they* fear: an optimized population of people who are awake and unified. Healthy people are very difficult to control.

PRIMAL WISDOM

It is not the critic who counts; not the man who points out how the strong man stumbles, or where the doer of deeds could have done them better. The credit belongs to the man who is actually in the arena, whose face is marred by dust and sweat and blood; who strives valiantly; who errs, who comes up short again and again, because there is no effort without error and shortcoming; but who does actually strive to do the deeds; who knows great enthusiasms, the great devotions; who spends himself in a worthy cause; who at the best knows in the end the triumph of high achievement, and who at the worst, if he fails, at least fails while daring greatly, so that his place shall never be with those cold and timid souls who neither know victory nor defeat.
—THEODORE ROOSEVELT

The Price of Fear

The United States was founded on the principle that it was worth taking a giant risk to achieve independence. Our founding fathers were surely scared of leaving the safety of the structure they knew, even one controlled by a power-hungry and ruthless monarch. Not everyone agreed with them. Many shouted that they had to stay captives because it was safer, that they couldn't possibly govern themselves. That risk, defiance, and effort to achieve freedom caused a revolution and was the basis for the creation of the United States.

Now, a couple of hundred years later, we find ourselves in a similar position. We need to trust ourselves to be free to make our own decisions, apart from what the power structures would like us to do. But that's scary. We get it. Trusting yourself and taking responsibility for your own actions and your own life means that whatever you do is on you. If you live according to what someone else tells you, you have the illusion that you are no longer responsible for your life. You're free to blame others for your unhappiness or the conditions of your life, but that also means you have outsourced your power, and that's exactly what they want. That's why they keep you in fear.

Fear is a powerful control mechanism. Here are some of the ways the power structures use it to keep us under their control:

1. **They undermine** our physical and mental health until we feel too insecure to fully understand our situation and make our own decisions. They plant seeds of doubt in our minds so we stop trusting ourselves.

2. **They indoctrinate** us with the notion that we have a problem, only they have the solution, and the only way we can have access to the solution is to do and believe what they say.

3. **They separate** us from each other, so we feel isolated and alone. They convince us that digital communication is better and easier than actual physical proximity. They tell us that what is different, unfamiliar, and foreign is also dangerous. They divide us to conquer us.

4. **They scare** us by telling us that if we don't let them protect us, our basic needs are at risk. They exaggerate threats to safety and security, convincing us that the world is a dangerous place. Killer storms! Alien invasions! Murder hornets!

5. **They moralize,** creating arbitrary descriptions of what is right and wrong that do not coincide with what most people consider to be right and wrong based on their internal compass. They convince people that those who fit their description of morality are good and those who don't are bad.

6. **They polarize** by encouraging black-and-white thinking and denying complexity. There is good and evil, and all people and things are either one or the other, with no in-between. They reward people for taking sides against each other on the most minor issues.

7. **They incite** by encouraging aggression and hate against those who have different beliefs, different skin colors, different accents, different traditions, and different lifestyles than the "norm."

These techniques are well known and familiar to those who are in power, as well as those who study human behavior. Edward Bernays, nephew to Sigmund Freud, is called the "father of public relations" (he was responsible for changing the concept of propaganda into the concept of public relations). He was fascinated by the idea that human behavior is driven by irrational force and that by understanding culture, behavior could be manipulated without the knowledge of those being manipulated. He used this knowledge to become a successful marketer.

One famous client of his was the American Tobacco Company, whose executives came to him because they wanted to tap a new market for their product—they wanted to sell cigarettes to women. In 1929, it was considered taboo for women to smoke in public, so Bernays consulted with one of his uncle's protégés, A. A. Brill, to find out what cigarettes represented to women. The answer: male power. So, Bernays created a campaign called "Torches of Freedom," to convince women that smoking would free them from the bondage of a patriarchal society. A "Torches of Freedom Parade" on Fifth Avenue in New York City made national news, as young women eagerly gathered (not knowing the health risks) to smoke Lucky Strikes in public. Women have been buying cigarettes ever since, to the delight of Big Tobacco. Of course, smoking didn't do anything to free women from male power. All it really did was put women at greater risk of lung cancer, but the campaign was a huge success.

Another Bernays victory was to convince the American public that bacon and eggs was a good breakfast to sell more bacon. (Incidentally, we agree that bacon and eggs is an excellent breakfast, but that's not the point here.) At the time, people mostly ate light breakfasts of toast and juice, but in his 1928 book *Propaganda,* he wrote that he consulted doctors to get their opinion about whether it was better to eat a light breakfast or a hearty breakfast. Most doctors said a hearty breakfast was preferable, so Bernays leveraged his "doctor-approved" hearty breakfast of bacon and eggs to sway public opinion, changing the face of American breakfasts for decades to come.

This is how easy to manipulate people are. If it's "doctor-approved" (or if "experts believe," "studies say," or "everybody knows"), we'd better run off and do it, buy it, or believe it. If it will "give you more power" or "make you healthier," then we're all in, without ever asking what the doctors actually said (they didn't mention eggs or bacon), or whether that thing in question—that idea, product, fad, cigarette—will actually give us power, health, or anything else we want. Will it give power to somebody else—namely, whoever is profiting? Maybe it actually will benefit you (like those bacon and eggs), and maybe it won't, but advertising isn't going to give you the true or complete story either way.

To break free, ask questions. Doubt. Be discerning. Don't be gullible. Asking questions is the first step to freedom from manipulation and control.

So ask yourself: Who are the zookeepers?

PRIMAL UPRISING LITMUS TEST

> Who profits from it?
> Does it empower you, or does it empower someone else?
> Does it keep you safe, or does it keep you caged?
> Does it support your opinion, or does it support the truth?
> Does it make you afraid? Is the fear justified?

2

WHO OWNS THE ZOO?

Whatever happened to having a healthy distrust of authority? When did we lose our skepticism and suspicion? Have we forgotten that they too are mere mortals? Have we forgotten how to think for ourselves and how to take responsibility for our own lives?

—Patrick Carroll, Canadian writer

If we are all in a human zoo, who owns the zoo? Who are the zookeepers? We call them the Bigs, and they are powerful, insidious, and in control. They are the power structures that have grown up within our society—mostly composed of white men, by the way—that were originally useful, but that now have more influence than what was ever intended by those who founded them. They are primarily motivated by profit rather than the best interest of the people. They keep us all captive, psychologically if not physically. They control not just in obvious ways but in subtle ways, and understanding them is essential to understanding the nature of our captivity and the necessity for our escape.

Although we could break them down into many smaller categories, there are seven primary Bigs that are the essential threats to human health, happiness, and freedom. They are:

25

1. Big Ag
2. Big Pharma
3. Big Medical
4. Big Business
5. Big Government
6. Big Military
7. Big Banking

The Bigs are complexly and often opaquely connected, working together in mutually beneficial ways to profit from the people who operate under their control. And we let them do it! We let Big Ag and Big Government manage our diets, and Big Medical and Big Pharma manage our health. We let Big Business manage our careers, and Big Media and Big Tech (part of Big Business) manage our attention. We let Big Government tax us for working and charge us for social security and tell us what we can and can't do, and we let Big Banking manage our entire financial system, including our own money, at every conceivable level.

We have outsourced most of our lives and most of our power to the Bigs, and most people don't realize it. It's just "how things are," but to truly understand how controlled you are in your own life by the Bigs, let's get to know them better. Know thy enemy! We don't know everything about them, and that is on purpose. We can only guess that if we knew everything they were doing, we would all stand up and say, "Wait a minute . . . who thought this was a good idea?!" Here's what we do know (with a healthy dose of our own perspective thrown in).

Don't Buy into the Bigs

The Bigs have transformed from once-useful institutions into a seven-headed, profit-motivated hydra that keeps growing as it feeds on power and control. Let's dive down and have a look at what they're doing right in front of us. Watch out, Bigs! We have our eyes on you.

Big Ag

In the human zoo, our food may as well be "human chow," dumped in front of us for us to pay for and consume, like it or not. We have the illusion of food freedom when what we actually have is food tyranny. We think we choose what to eat, but we are manipulated into thinking we want food that doesn't nourish us, and our choices are limited beyond what most of us know.

Big Ag includes the food giants like Nestlé, PepsiCo, Coca-Cola, Tyson, Mars, Archer-Daniels-Midland, Cargill, Dannon, Kellogg's, General Mills, Conagra, and more. It is also intimately linked to the United States Food and Drug Administration (FDA) and Department of Agriculture (USDA). It profits from food sales, and many of this industry's leaders have advised and continue to advise the government on what it should tell people to eat.

The government subsidizes (pays farmers to grow) cheap crops— wheat to be made into refined flour, soy to be made into protein isolates for processed food, and corn, which is mostly made to feed livestock (although it's not their natural diet) and to mix with gasoline to make cheap fuel. The small percentage of corn humans consume is primarily made into high-fructose corn syrup. These are the very foods that make us sick, fat, and lazy . . . and that make Big Ag so profitable. Our government hasn't banned many foods that contain additives, hormones, drugs, growth enhancers, artificial colors, and chemical preservatives that are banned almost everywhere else in the world, because they increase profits.

Meanwhile, they tax and penalize small farmers producing grass-fed and pastured meat and organic vegetables, driving up the cost of real whole food. The cheap products are priced well below their cost (because of subsidies), so they may be the only affordable foods for some people. But real, whole, organic food? No way. It's just not profitable. There is no Big Kale.

Our land was once covered in rich, fertile soil, constantly rejuvenated and regenerated by tens of millions of bison grazing and fertilizing and "tilling" it with their hooves. They roamed the plains from the Dakotas all the way down to Mexico, back and forth. The breadbasket of the US and its rich topsoil was built because of the bison. But we killed most of them, decimating a source of food that could have fed millions, and we've farmed the "breadbasket" nearly to death. Erosion and agricultural chemicals have all but destroyed the once diverse and nutrient-rich soil microbiome.

ROBB WOLF SAYS . . .

Our friend Robb Wolf, a former research biochemist who's now a paleo expert and co-author of *Sacred Cow: The Case for (Better) Meat* and other great books, is a champion of the bison:

> A crack team of NASA scientists couldn't, if they tried, design a more miraculous entity than the cow or bison. They convert sunlight, water, grass, and soil into highly nutritious, bio-available protein and fat, even while nurturing and regenerating the very land they graze on.

Today, rather than growing the diverse and nutrient-rich crops we could be growing and working to regenerate our soil, millions of acres of land are devoted primarily to just four heavily subsidized crops: corn, soy, wheat, and cotton. This is monoculture. Farmers that are getting subsidies grow these crops in rotation, which does nothing to regenerate the soil. There is almost ubiquitous use of the herbicide glyphosate (sold under the trade name Roundup) on these crops, despite the many studies showing that it is toxic and carcinogenic.[1] They use it over and over, year after year, on crop after crop. Then they feed those glyphosate-laden grains to us.

Big Ag is not Big Ag in a vacuum. Big Business runs the corporations that constitute Big Ag, and Big Government makes the mandates that regulate Big Ag (or don't), but in ways that prioritize profit over human and environmental health.

Consider that the agricultural company formerly known as Monsanto—manufacturer of Roundup—is one of the biggest names in Big Ag. They are now owned by Bayer (the pharmaceutical company that bought Monsanto for $66 billion in 2018). Bayer retired the notorious name "Monsanto" and took control, with the blessing of both US and European regulators.

Think about the implications of this move. It's no small thing that this was allowed to happen. Big Pharma running Big Ag? Talk about a conflict of interest—"Let's make food that makes people sick so they have to buy more drugs!" It's thinly veiled corruption at a level beyond common knowledge. And by the way, it was Monsanto (along with Dow Chemical and Diamond Shamrock) that manufactured Agent Orange,[2] the herbicide used so lethally in Vietnam. They have never paid a cent for their crimes against humanity with the use of those bioweapons. A company heavily involved in pharmaceuticals that owns a chemical company heavily involved in food production that can also make bioweapons? It may sound like a conspiracy theory, but it's not simply a theory. Don't believe us? Go look for yourself. We're just relaying information. It's out there for anyone to see.

Most people don't pay attention to the laws that are passed involving this high level of agricultural, chemical, pharmaceutical, and military deal-making. Most people don't have the time, and honestly, most people probably really don't want to know. It's easier to stay safely ignorant. The problem is that you are not safe. Not safe at all. People don't usually realize this until something happens to a loved one (like a chemical poisoning from a local water supply—the tragedy in Flint, Michigan, comes to mind[3]). Only then do they start digging.

How do we bring down such a powerful and entrenched system? It's already happening to some extent. There are whispers and murmurs and localized action, but it rarely reaches across state lines. For a discussion of some of the exciting grassroots efforts to decentralize the food system, see chapter 20.

Big Pharma

There is a pill for every problem, or so it seems. How many people do you know who aren't on a single medication? That's because Big Pharma profits from pharmaceutical drugs and controls what drugs we have access to, and they are good at working with Big Business (via Big Media and Big Tech) to convince us that we need their products. When Big Pharma needs a new market, all they have to do is make one up (fidgety kids? moody women? people who eat junk food and get constipated?), then find or make a drug to "fix" the "problem."

We are the only country that allows pharmaceutical companies to advertise directly to consumers. See an advertisement on TV about a medication for depression, heartburn, erectile dysfunction, or whatever, and you can "ask your doctor" about it. A pharmaceutical rep has already prepped the doctor for your questions. The doctor prescribes the drug. The patient feels like the doctor listened, the doctor feels like the patient is satisfied, and the pharmaceutical company makes a profit. It sounds like a win-win-win, but it's only a win for Big Pharma. None of it has anything to do with *your health.*

PRIMAL WISDOM

Science advances one funeral at a time.
—MAX PLANCK

The FDA is Big Pharma's primary mouthpiece, which is disturbing since it is supposed to be a regulatory agency, not a shill for pharmaceutical profiteering. Big Pharma is intimately associated with the insurance industry as well as Big Ag and Big Business. They also provide a substantial share of the funding for the education of medical professionals[4] (a conflict of interest, to be sure). This model of healthcare was set up in a time when the primary threat to health was infectious disease. Now, the primary threat to health is chronic disease, and chronic disease is not something best treated by conventional medical intervention. It's almost always best treated—and, ideally, prevented—with lifestyle intervention. But that's not profitable.

Why aren't we asking why people need these drugs? Why do people have failing health? What are they eating? How much sleep are they getting? How often are they exercising? How do they feel about their relationships? What is causing them stress?

It may be easier to pop a pill than answer these questions, but it's certainly not in your best interest (you might need that medication, but you can still ask the questions). The sad reality is that you are a profit center to these entities and nothing more. It's an unsavory idea, but once we come to terms with it, everything else begins to make more sense.

WHAT ABOUT VACCINES?

We aren't "anti-vaxxers," but we believe in discerning vaccinations. Isn't it interesting that you can't sue a pharmaceutical company for damages done due to negative effects from vaccines?[5] Isn't it interesting that they already have taxpayer money set aside to cover the damage from vaccines they already know will occur? Why are the taxpayers covering this liability when it's Big Pharma that stands to make billions? And why aren't they held accountable when something goes wrong? If you need a vaccine, if the benefits to public health are proven and the risks are minimal, we support it, but those facts should be available to us. Without transparency, Big Pharma can do whatever it wants.

Big Medical

Ideally, nobody should need healthcare unless they get severely injured or have a life-threatening infection or rare disease—but how profitable would that be? Big Medical is what we call the "sick-care" system that includes hospital systems, insurance companies, and medical schools. It is in league with Big Pharma as well as Big Ag because both contribute to feeding Big Medical its customers. Poor food leads to illness, which leads to medical care, which leads to prescriptions.

Our bodies and their intelligent and capable immune systems should be our primary source of healing. Yet, here we are. According to the Pentagon, 71 percent of the 34 million seventeen- to twenty-four-year-olds in the US would not qualify for military service due to health and educational limitations.[6] Millennials are the largest generation alive today, but their health has been declining and is generally worse than their parents'.[7] We aren't doing a very good job at preventing chronic disease.

Unfortunately, prevention isn't Big Medical's concern. It's not that doctors don't want to focus on wellness. They just aren't trained for it. They are also under licensure pressure, liability pressure, and pressure to meet quotas for procedures. They have to march to the tune of huge hospital systems, university systems, and insurance companies, and that means keeping you in need of the system. Doctors are strongly incentivized to make decisions that are not in your best interest, nor in theirs.

We have friends who say, "It's not true! Doctors are good-hearted. They are healers. They wouldn't try to keep you sick. They took an oath!" We agree that most individual doctors are good-hearted and really do want to help people, but unfortunately, doctors' hands are tied. We know more than a few doctors who left the profession because they were not allowed to practice medicine in a way they felt was right, ethical, and patient-centric.

Alternative medicine seeks to go against this grain and we know many great functional, integrative, and other holistic doctors and health providers who work tirelessly to champion health care instead of sick care. We love them, but Big Medical doesn't. Big Medical constantly works (via Big Media and Big Government regulation) to discredit any form of healthcare that could cut into their profits. Many ethical and effective alternative practitioners have been censored on social media or have been otherwise undermined, or even sued, when they say publicly that wellness, self-care, and healthy lifestyle practices could be useful in staving off a virus, supporting the immune system, or preventing chronic conditions like heart disease or cancer.

Hey, we get that nobody should coerce people into treatments that are dangerous or that keep them from getting treatments that will actually help them, but shouldn't you get to choose whether or not to buy into someone's healthcare advice? In an unfettered free market of ideas, it should be up to each person to sift through the information and come to their own decisions about their own health. Do your due diligence and find out for yourself whether someone has the training and experience to help you. Follow the money to find the truth.

Big Business

Our so-called capitalist country is slowly devolving into a dictatorship or an oligarchy with a drone economy. The free market is no longer free—we've transitioned to a rigged, "cabalistic" one, without most of us noticing it happened. Big business is not just about making money anymore. It's about amassing power, and money is a means to power for the few.

Big Business is composed of the largest corporations and the most powerful billionaires (again, mostly white men)—the 1 percent. They include Big Media and Big Tech as well as corporate lobbyists and the US Stock Exchange, which links Big Business with Big Banking. Big Business has its hands in Big Medical, Big Pharma, and Big Ag, and their bottom line depends on getting your attention. Big Tech companies like Google, Facebook, Apple, and Amazon are the interfaces through which people buy and know almost everything these days. They are the biggest entities on the planet right now, with the most unbridled control, and money is both their incentive and motive. They have studied you and they know how to get you to see what they want you to see and buy what they show you.

How do you compete, with your mom-and-pop business, your freelance gigs, or your little start-up, when Big Business not only can afford to offer things cheaper but also has the leverage to control everyone's attention? There will be a ceiling, and it will be low, and you will not easily be able to break through it. If you somehow manage to, and you threaten the profit of those in power, you can bet your little business isn't going to survive for very long—that is, unless you decide to go over to the side of the Bigs. That's what we call cartel capitalism.

We would never begrudge a business from making a profit, but we also believe profit shouldn't be at the expense of the health and well-being of humans (corporations are not humans, no matter what Big Government says!). Business is business, but there also have to be checks and balances so profit doesn't come before people.

We can say, "There should be government oversight!" but the problem is that government oversight inevitably ends up being influenced by lobbyists and money. We don't want government oversight. Give *us* the oversight so we can free the market, free our attention, and decentralize Big Business.

In chapter 20, we'll talk more about what a decentralized business model would look like, and how it is already happening, with the rise of the gig economy.

PRIMAL WISDOM

Where the people fear the government, you have tyranny.
Where the government fears the people, you have liberty.
—JOHN BASIL BARNHILL

Big Government

Big Government includes all the branches of the US government at the national level, and the governments of the major world economies at the international level. They are connected to all the other Bigs through the influential work of lobbyists, special interest groups, and Big Government, which controls international trade, as well as the highly profitable regulation (that is, taxing) of things like alcohol, tobacco, and firearms. Big Government profits off you by taxing you for working and for owning things, via the IRS. They keep track of people covertly, via the alphabet soup of covert agencies: the FBI, CIA, NSA, DEA, DIA, the Department of Homeland Security, the Space Force, and all the other intelligence branches of the US military.

There was a time in our lives when we thought politics were fun. Those were the good old days! Keith was a poli-sci major in college and Michelle used to be a campaign manager for a senate race. We enjoyed being in the thick of the debates, immersing ourselves in the ideology and the philosophy. Then it got to the point that everywhere we looked, we saw corruption.

It's pretty clear that our political system isn't working very well anymore. We think the two-party system is part of the problem because the two parties are really just two sides of the same coin. There may be a big difference between how they publicly express what they want, but it's all a show, and we've bought into the lie. Both the Republican and Democratic parties work together to keep the system going, to keep the profits flowing. Much like the way the NFC and the AFC both "work" for the profit of the NFL, there is no game without manufactured rivalry and competition. Everybody wants to root for their side, but when your team comes before the welfare of the country, we've got a problem.

Remember that one of the most powerful ways to control people is to divide and conquer by inducing fear and disdain of "the other." This is exactly what a two-party system does. Why do you think they make us choose? Because then we fight among ourselves and stay angry and divided and afraid of "them" because they are not like "us."

Another part of this problem is that because of the corruption endemic to the system, we always seem to be faced with two poor options—two corrupt options, even if some of them hide it better than others. Two options nobody really wants to make. It's common to hear people say they are voting for "the lesser of two evils." People frequently vote against someone, not for someone. Why aren't we voting for the best candidates for the position? Why do we settle for "least bad" when we should be given "best"? Because truly capable, honest candidates with the best interest of people as their priority aren't usually corrupt enough to do what it takes to achieve that national stage. You can find some good people in politics, but they don't usually get very far. Just as good doctors have to operate within a corrupt system, so do many of those who run for office. The system is specifically designed to keep itself running, and that means it is stacked against anyone getting elected who will disrupt the system in any meaningful way.[8]

Big Military

Big Business, Big Government, and Big Military: it's an unholy trinity. Big Military involves all the US armed forces, which are closely tied to the defense industry (Big Guns? Big Bombs?), which manufactures and profits from the sale of military products. There are a handful of defense companies that produce all the goods for war—every bullet, every bomb, every jet fighter, every aircraft carrier, all of it. They are incentivized to support war because without war, they would go out of business. You can't make money making bombs if nobody is trying to bomb anything.

President Dwight D. Eisenhower predicted what was to come after World War II. In his farewell address, he famously said:

> In the councils of government, we must guard against the acquisition of unwarranted influence, whether sought or unsought, by the military-industrial complex. The potential for the disastrous rise of misplaced power exists and will persist. We must never let the weight of this combination endanger our liberties or democratic processes. We should take nothing for granted. Only an alert and knowledgeable citizenry can compel the proper meshing of the huge industrial and military machinery of defense with our peaceful methods and goals, so that security and liberty may prosper together.

He tried to warn us, but our citizenry has been neither alert nor knowledgeable about what has been happening, and now we are exactly where he feared we might be. For generations, we have been lulled into inaction (and not by accident) by "bread and circuses"—distractions and superficial entertainment to keep us happy and docile and oblivious to what's really going on. As the Wizard of Oz said: "Pay no attention to the man behind the curtain!"

The military-industrial complex didn't come about overnight. It was incremental, and no one said anything. We didn't vote with our attention, or with our dollars, or with our actual votes in the voting booth, against small legal (and illegal) shifts—one little adjustment to a regulation here, one shift in a strategy there, one little "letting something slide"—until one day we woke up and realized that holy shit, we have no idea what's going on behind closed doors, who's planning what, or when we might suddenly find ourselves at war, just because it's profitable for the Bigs.

Big Banking

Most people probably think of banking as its own thing, apart from the other Bigs, but everything goes through the banks. They underlie all the other Bigs since the whole system runs on money. This one is the most secretive and most powerful Big of them all, an elite class of money handlers working the strings on the rest of the Bigs like some malevolent puppeteer.

When you consider the corporate structure inherent to our way of life, it all comes back to money. Our debt-ridden government is beholden to Big Banking. Our tax dollars go into Big Banking, and then the banks loan this money back to the government for infrastructure, at such a high rate that we can never, ever hope to pay it back. That is where our deficit comes from.[9]

It really amounts to money laundering and would technically be illegal, but it's been going on for so long that everybody accepts it. Meanwhile, Big Banking creates money out of thin air. There is no longer any gold standard—no precious metals or anything real to back it up. It's fiat currency. It's all smoke and mirrors. (If you really want to dive down a rabbit hole someday, look up "fractional reserve lending." We bet you'll come back up saying "WTF!")

Another aspect of Big Banking is its lending practices, which are set up against the individual, to benefit the Bigs. This is why the housing market crash happened in 2008, during which, as we've told you, the two of us lost almost everything. That crisis was the pinnacle of corruption—the lenders responsible for the housing crisis broke every rule when it comes to business banking, and the most powerful of them were never punished in any meaningful way. Their argument, when they asked to be bailed out of that trillion-plus-dollar mess? "We're too big to fail." Consider the irony of the leaders of those companies flying to Washington in their private jets to testify. "Bail us out with your taxpayer money even though we already screwed you over on your mortgages. If you don't bail us out, the whole country will collapse." It was all BS. We were collapsing anyway.

Right now, there is nothing to prevent such a crisis from happening again. Big Banking just turned around, waited a little bit of time, then put all the same structures in place. The last time was a wake-up call, but instead of asking how it happened, we just went back to business as usual.

• • •

Are you as angry as we are? Confused? Shaking your head in disbelief? Us, too. What kind of world do you want to live in? The zookeepers might be the FDA, or the USDA, or Bayer, or Pfizer, or the CDC, or the American Medical Association, or Amazon, or Apple, or Walmart, or the IRS, or the White House, or the FDIC, or whoever tells us we need an opaque power structure to oversee us and an authorized representative to tell us what we need, what we want, and what we think.

We say: "No." We say: "Enough." It's going to take some doing, and we're not going to tear it down overnight, but we do know that we can all start dismantling the bars of our cages now.

The good news is that people are already doing just that. The uprising has begun. You can be a part of that change. It starts with you, your family, your neighbors, your friends, your communities, and on up from the grass-roots to the glass ceiling—and right through it.

It's your decision. Are you willing to outsource those food, drug, health, business, government, and military decisions to somebody else? Or are you willing to actually look this whole nightmarish scenario in the eye so you can see what's really going on?

Pay attention. Ask questions. Rise up. You don't have to be a zoo animal, oblivious to what the zookeepers are doing. Don't let them tell you that asking questions and questioning authority is unpatriotic. It's the most patriotic thing you can do for your country. As Edmund Burke once said, "The only thing necessary for the triumph of evil is for good men to do nothing." When we act together, as a unified force, no Big can stand in our way. Together, we will be even Bigger.

PRIMAL UPRISING LITMUS TEST

> Is this food good for me, or only good for the person selling it to me?
> Does this medication or treatment address the "why," or only mask the symptoms?
> Who profits if I believe this, do this, buy this, or take this advice?
> Who is trying to capture my attention?
> What are the objectives of my leaders? Are they profit-motivated or people-motivated?
> Who wants my money, and how are they trying to get it?

3

YOUR ESCAPE PLAN

In captivity, one loses every way of acting over little details which satisfy the essentials of life. Everything has to be asked for: permission to go to the toilet, permission to ask a guard something, permission to talk to another hostage—to brush your teeth, use toilet paper, everything is a negotiation.

—Íngrid Betancourt, politician imprisoned in
Colombia for activism

Are you ready for your basic training, so we can rally the troops and unite the tribe against the insidious forces that are the Bigs? Are you ready to begin the process of conditioning for your ultimate escape from the human zoo? To live truly free means to possess optimal health, and in our world, that means we must optimize each of the seven pillars of health. Here is what we will be working on with you throughout this book.

The Seven Pillars of Health

Health isn't just not being sick. Health is a mind-body-spirit proposition. It is a whole-person, whole-life condition, and it starts with the physical but goes much further than that. These are the seven pillars of health:

1. **Physical health:** Through the foods you eat, the way you move, how well you sleep, and how you live, you build physical health, not just according to minimum requirements but for optimization.
2. **Mental health:** To escape from the human zoo, you need to be sharp, quick-thinking, good at problem solving, and also rational, contemplative, discerning, and creative.
3. **Emotional health:** To be fully aware of and willing to experience the entire range of human emotions is to be emotionally intelligent enough that you cannot be manipulated by fear.
4. **Spiritual health:** Without a sense of something higher than the individual, something worth believing in and fighting for, you cannot be a fully whole and healthy person.
5. **Financial health:** Financial health is about resources, abundance, and understanding that money isn't good or bad—it's energy.
6. **Relational health:** Human connection is perhaps our most challenging and also our most fulfilling duty and honor in this lifetime.
7. **Tribal health:** Humans are designed to operate in tribes, because we are greater in numbers than the sum of our parts.

These seven pillars represent the environmental crucible in which we evolved, but as our society has become more complex and its power structures more opaque, those pillars have been crumbling. As we described in the previous chapter, a sick, tired, foggy, diverted, distracted, and divided population is easy to control.

To lay the groundwork for the work to come, let's set the scene.

Rat Park

In the 1970s, psychologist Bruce Alexander conducted a now-famous study often referred to as "Rat Park." Its original purpose was to study addiction. Dr. Alexander knew that when rats were put alone in cages with two water bottles—one with plain water and one laced with cocaine or heroin—the rats would choose the drugs and dose themselves until they died. Dr. Alexander wondered if the drugs were the real appeal, or if the environments the rats lived in were affecting their behavior. After all, rats in the wild (even if "the wild" is a sewer in a big city) are never alone in a box.

So Dr. Alexander built what he called Rat Park. It was a large enclosure filled with lots of things for rats to do, along with a community of rats that could interact with each other. The rats could explore, exercise, breed, engage in mental challenges, even "argue" and squabble.

We bet you can guess what happened: The rats flourished, and as Dr. Alexander suspected would happen, they hardly ever chose the drugged water over the plain water. When they did, it was infrequent, and none of them ever overdosed.[10]

When it comes to captivity, we aren't much different than those rats. We are meant to live in physical contact with other people, move and challenge ourselves, learn and play and think and exercise our emotions. We are meant to eat real whole food, and be outside during the day. We are meant to support each other and interact with each other, work out our differences, and create communities. We are meant to live natural lives, closer to the way our Paleolithic ancestors lived, rather than sitting all day staring at and communicating through screens without much physical effort or face-to-face engagement. Living in interactive communities with healthy food and movement, allowed to pursue our passions and develop our skills and know we are contributing to the greater good is the kind of life that makes people happy.

Of course, this is all much more complex than what rats need because we are more complex than rats, but the basic idea is the same: Give us what we need to live our lives the way we were built to live them, and we will enjoy our lives more. We will be healthier. We will thrive. Today, we are both blessed and cursed with the ability to create our own environments, but because the modern world is mismatched to our ancient physiology, we don't always know how to create those environments in our own best interest.

KYLE KINGSBURY SAYS . . .

Our friend Kyle Kingsbury is a retired mixed martial artist and the host of the *Kyle Kingsbury Podcast*. Here's what he reminds us about owning our own health:

We've been lied to about our health since before we were born. We have placed our power in the hands of an establishment that doesn't understand what health is. We bow to the unhealthy in a white lab coat. Your personal sovereignty is your responsibility. The knowledge and excellence of your body must be your passion. The body is a tuning fork to all levels of awareness, peace, and health. If you wish to know thyself, the body is the foundational key to all inner knowing.

Optimal Foraging Theory

For the vast majority of human history, we operated under what science calls *optimal foraging theory*. This theory suggests that every living entity tries to get the maximum amount of nutrition and energy with the minimum amount of energy expenditure. For most of human history, food required a lot of energy to procure. Not knowing when our next meal would be, we had to get our calories wherever we could and conserve them for as long as we could. Otherwise, we might starve. Humans used to be largely nomadic, so movement was necessarily for survival, to find food, escape danger, and follow the herds. This kept us fit and alert, but whenever movement was optional, humans generally chose not to do it because, again, we had to conserve our calories and energy for when we really needed it—to run from a predator or run after prey. We share this with most living beings. Whether you are a bacterium or a lion, tiger, or bear, you will live according to this basic principle of survival.

In addition to prioritizing rest, humans hunted animals with the highest fat content and foraged plants with the highest nutrient content and medicinal value (like leafy greens and certain herbs) or energy content (like sweet fruits and starchy root vegetables). Nature, in turn, complied with this need: Animals that are fatter are not as fleet afoot as animals that are leaner, so they are easier to bring down—and they are at their fattest when we needed them the most, just before a long winter. Sweeter fruits fall from the trees, bushes, and vines in the fall when we too must fatten up for the cold season, while greens, roots, and tubers are easy to gather throughout the spring and summer when we need less fat but also need to replenish our nutrient stores.

This is why it feels so good to eat high-calorie food, and it doesn't always feel good to exert ourselves. It goes against an instinct that is no longer relevant to our lives but is still deeply ingrained. It takes an unusual human being to choose to move without a payoff. Those modern payoffs may not be about survival. They might be about winning a game, beating a personal best, or looking good naked. But while all these things can be motivating, they don't feel urgent. Telling the average person that they should move because it's "healthy" is a very tough sell, and willpower is a limited resource.

Working directly in opposition to ancient instincts is our modern environment. Now we can easily acquire foods rich in calories, especially that irresistible combination of sugar, salt, and fat. We don't have to hunt for French fries and cupcakes (and food companies know this and take advantage of it for profit). Highly palatable foods are extremely hard to exist, and often come with a side of industrial chemicals and highly refined oils, sweeteners, and grains. If these foods were wild-caught game and wild leafy greens, that would at least be nutrient-rich, but instead, our food is artificially colored and preserved and wrapped in plastic. It's zoo food. It's like the processed chow they give rats or monkeys or dogs—but worse because at least those foods are scientifically formulated to nourish, rather than to exploit a built-in human vulnerability.

Meanwhile, remember that instinct to conserve energy? We're lucky that we don't have to run after predators anymore, but what are we conserving our energy for? To walk to the refrigerator? To drive to the grocery store? To warm up a meal in the microwave or run on a treadmill at a gym? We don't have to walk anywhere. We can drive. We sit all day. We don't have to chase our food. Our lives our physically and calorically easy. Too easy.

Many of us believe that this mismatch is the primary reason why we have the highest levels of chronic disease ever recorded, but, seeing where we are is the beginning of changing where we're going. If we acknowledge our current predicament, then we at least know the rules of the game. The human zoo is like a casino: the house always wins. If you don't know that, you'll probably lose. If you do, at least you have a chance.

The Natural Human Environment

What we really need is a natural environment for humans—our own version of Rat Park. To figure out what that might look like, we can consult what we know by looking back, way back, to when we lived more natural lives. That time in human history, before we had computers, cars, modern medicine, or agriculture, holds important clues for what we need to reclaim our health. What would we be eating and doing "in the wild"? What would our environments look like?

First, we evolved in an environment where movement was imperative and food was hunted or gathered. We were (and still are) obligate movers and opportunistic eaters. We flourished because we had metabolic flexibility and could ingest and utilize just about anything we could get our hands on. Humans can survive on just about any natural diet and in just about any natural environment. Consider the Inuit, who ate mostly seafood and fat, as well as things you can't get in the grocery store, like fermented whale meat, fish heads, and seal flippers. They had to contend with subzero temperatures and a climate of snow and ice, with very little access to plant food. Even so, they were active, healthy, and almost never obese.

Contrast that to South America or New Guinea, where hunter-gatherers ate mostly fruit and starchy roots and tubers with very little meat, and lived in a climate that was lush, tropical, and hot. They also had very little obesity, and chronic diseases like heart disease and cancer were virtually nonexistent.

To get a glimpse of a natural human existence now, consider the Hadza tribe, a modern hunter-gatherer society living in northern Tanzania. They have a high infant mortality rate, but if they survive hazardous infancy and childhood, then make it through the dangerous younger years of their teens and twenties (when they might die from an infectious disease or an accident), they typically live as long as we do.[11] They eat mostly fruit with some starchy tubers and small animals, and they too are very rarely over-weight and almost never die from chronic diseases, even when they live into their seventies or beyond. They mostly die from the same things we died from in this country before we had access to emergency medical care and antibiotics.

Natural diets, time outside, moving all day long, and depending on each other for survival are all important core characteristics of the natu-ral human environment. Each person has their role: hunting or gathering, preparing food, taking care of children, building shelters, making clothes, or protecting the tribe from an outside threat. Each one of them matters, and the group matters most of all. Their togetherness is an essential part of their lives.

This is an often-forgotten part of ancient existence: tribe. We need each other on an emotional level, even when we don't need each other for physical survival. Humans can literally die of loneliness. Disturbing exper-iments in which baby animals or even human infants were raised without physical contact have had tragic consequences. We are programmed to be together—not isolated in cubicles, staring at screens, or forming relation-ships with characters in computer games or on television shows.

In many ways, we've got it easy, with our climate-controlled environ-ments, physically easy lives, easily accessible foods, and digital communi-cation, but at what price? The Paleo f(x) motto is: *Challenge Authority, Defy Dogma, Demand Different.* We challenge you to consider how you were meant to live. How does that differ from what the Bigs tell you to eat and do, buy and think? We challenge you to defy dogma by questioning the status quo and looking for your own answers about how you were meant to live. We challenge you to demand different—better food, more movement, more understanding, discernment, connection.

How can we best leverage what we know about our human history to advance into an evolved human future that is more paradise than hellscape? We believe that we can eat a natural diet and practice natural movement and reclaim natural relationships without sacrificing those technological advancements that make living in this age so thrilling, not to mention convenient. That is the essence of our vision of paleo: Looking to the past in order to move more successfully into the future. How we do that, friends and fellow tribespeople, should be entirely up to us.

Change the Story

The human zoo is a story. The bars we stand behind are only as strong as we let them be. We have to be stronger, and that means we have to be healthy, from head to toe and inside to outside. True survival isn't survival of the fittest. It's survival of the most adaptable and resilient. That's what you're going to become. Let's set confusion and fear aside. Let's set transferring responsibility onto our captors aside. Those are zoo conditions and zoo politics. When you change the narrative from "Human Zoo" to "Human Evolution," you can live in a better story.

Throughout the rest of this book, we're going to work on your health, tackling the seven pillars one at a time. Each section will contain information to inform you, words to inspire you, and actions you can take that will change you in meaningful ways. We'll give you things you can do right now, and things you can incorporate into your life long-term, along with plenty to think about. Unlike some health books that are written only to make you feel better or avoid disease, this book is about setting your mind and body free so you can take full advantage of that freedom to fulfill your purpose on Earth.

The freer you are, the less you will be dependent on anyone else for your survival or happiness. You won't even need this book! You might want to read it anyway, to consider our opinions and try our techniques and maybe join our tribe, and you are welcome! But you won't need us, and that is exactly what we want for you: to be so physically, mentally, emotionally, financially, relationally, and tribally strong that your life belongs to you and you love living it, in cooperation and collaboration with your tribe. This is how we will create a new world where everyone can become who they truly are, invest in their own gifts, and contribute to a better society. Let's evolve naturally into a future world where people—not dollars, not corporations, not Bigs—have sovereignty and control over their own lives again.

We think that's a future worth training for.

PRIMAL UPRISING LITMUS TEST

> Am I allowing my food choices to be hijacked by food companies, or am I eating a natural human diet?
> Am I moving because I can, or sitting because I can?
> Who has my attention?
> What kind of life do I want to live?
> Am I discerning enough to take wisdom from the past but still plan for the future?

PART II
THE PHYSICAL PILLAR

Man does not simply exist but always decides what his existence will be, what he will become the next moment. By the same token, every human being has the freedom to change at any instant.

—Viktor Frankl

4

FOOD FREEDOM

As for butter versus margarine, I trust cows more than chemists.

—Joan Gussow

In order to escape from the human zoo, you need to be healthy, and to be healthy, the most important thing you can do is get your food figured out. What you eat affects *everything else* about your health. This is the place to begin.

Your doctor may not ever ask about what you are eating. That's because most doctors (unless they are alternative practitioners) don't receive much if any training on nutrition. Even if they did advise you on diet, they probably don't have the information you need. You, however, can discover what you need to know on your own by exploring the natural human diet. Nobody counseled our distant ancestors on what to eat. Nature provided. That's where to start looking.

Paleo 2.0

There are a lot of misconceptions about the paleo diet. We've had a lot of people tell us that they could "never do paleo" because it's too hard, rigid, or expensive, but then when we ask them how they eat, they say things like, "I'm keto" or "I do Whole 30."

Both Keto and Whole 30 *are versions of paleo,* and both are more restrictive than looser versions of the paleo diet. Paleo can mean many things. It is broad and diverse, but people often don't realize this. Many people who are actually *doing the paleo diet* think they couldn't possibly follow it!

Another misconception is that paleo is basically "low carb and Cross-Fit." This (arguably) used to be true, or at least these were both popular choices for early adoptees of the paleo diet, and these are still viable choices for a paleo lifestyle, but they are not the only paths to paleo. CrossFit is certainly not a requirement for living a paleo lifestyle, and although most paleo diets are on the low-carb side, they certainly don't have to be.

Some people think the paleo diet is a carnivore diet, or that you have to eat raw meat and that you can't eat any vegetables—again, that can be one (extreme) version of paleo, but most people who follow the paleo diet eat huge amounts of vegetables, like our hunter-gatherer ancestors did. Some people think paleo is all about butter and bacon (viable paleo foods but not the only paleo foods) or that you can't eat fruit (you certainly can, although not everyone does) or that you can't eat a paleo diet and be a vegetarian (you can!), or that you can't ever let a grain, a bean, a cookie, or a cube of cheese pass your lips (fake news).

Maybe it's a PR issue, but paleo isn't a fad, it's not extreme, and it's certainly not unhealthy. Paleo, as it exists today, is flexible and customizable. A lot of the negative messaging comes from a system that profits from the sale of processed food and products that come from subsidized grain and soy crops (none of which are necessary foods for human health).

We want people to know that a natural human diet can change their health for the better, and to say otherwise is ridiculous. Health is both your right and your responsibility as a member of the human tribe, but we aren't going to nitpick about how to do that, beyond the primary message that real, whole food is the answer to optimized health and an optimized society. Sure, you *could* make your version of the paleo diet rigid or expensive, but it certainly doesn't have to be, and isn't for most of those who practice it. It certainly isn't for us.

A Diet for Free People

Even within our own household, we have different versions of the paleo diet. Keith's version of paleo is low in carbs, mostly grain-free and sugar-free, with a lot of healthy unsaturated fats and bioavailable proteins. This works with Keith's proclivity for exercise and lifting heavy things. He focuses on protein because he needs that muscle repair, but every now and then, he might eat some rice or sweet potatoes.

Michelle's version of paleo is a bit lower in fat, a bit higher in fruit, and focuses more on fiber and vegetables. This works best for Michelle's digestive health, hormonal balance, and genetics, which indicate that she may not process saturated fat efficiently. She can eat white potatoes, but sweet potatoes and rice make her blood sugar spike.

There are potentially as many other versions of paleo as there are people. A paleo diet can be made up of mostly (or solely) plant foods, or mostly (or solely) animal foods, but usually, there is a balance of both: lots of plants, lots of fiber, lots of nutrients, along with high-quality animal protein and fat. We don't think a vegan diet is the optimal diet for humans (it requires more pinpointed supplementation—more on that later), but if that is your preference, you can definitely be a paleo vegan. The only real "rule" is that most of the time, food should be natural and whole, not fake and processed. Processed food contains chemicals and preservatives that are known carcinogens, endocrine disruptors, and obesogens. There's nothing paleo about those!

How you "do paleo" depends on your preferences, your budget, and what is available. How strict you are about it depends on what you want to get from your diet. You might be going for weight loss or muscle gain or more energy, and those goals may all impact how you design your own diet.

There is no one-size-fits-all macronutrient ratio or exact food list. You can go low-carb, high-fat, lower-fat, or focus on plant fats. You can eliminate dairy, legumes, grains, and sugars, or just lighten up on your consumption. As long as you keep it real, focus on what works for you personally, and choose the highest-quality, most natural food you can find and afford, you can call yourself "paleo." That's the only aspect of nutrition that those of us in the Paleo 2.0-sphere really care about. The big picture is what matters. If you are making whole food decisions most of the time, you will notice profound physical (and mental) benefits. (Visit our Resources webpage at PrimalUprising.com/BookResources for sourcing on some of our favorite whole-food products, from olive oil to bison.)

PROCESSED *AND* PALEO?

Sometimes people ask us about processed foods labeled as paleo. Admittedly, it's kind of a contradiction in terms because packaged paleo bars, meat sticks, veggie chips, or dark chocolate squares are not whole foods. They are processed, although usually not nearly as much as more common junk foods, and they almost always contain much higher-quality ingredients. (Some of our favorite companies include Epic, Siete, Primal Kitchen, Evolved, and Coracao.) These exist because in the modern world, we don't always have time to cook. Higher quality packaged snacks are a way to compromise by championing small ethical companies making improvements to a food category that leaves much to be desired. If you're going to eat potato chips, they can be made from organic potatoes fried or baked in avocado oil. If you're going to eat chocolate, it can be 88 percent raw cacao. No processed food is as good as a bowl of berries or a sweet potato, but on the spectrum of pure to toxic, paleo snacks are on the right side of center.

Just remember that, whenever someone tells you that "paleo is impossible" or "there is no such thing as a paleo diet" or "that diet isn't healthy," it's not about reenacting caveman life. We can't eat the foods they ate anyway;

we no longer live in the same world, but we can make the best possible choices most of the time for health in an unhealthy world. And it all starts with food.

How to Start

When Keith was twelve years old, he signed up for a Thai kickboxing class. The teacher was one of the last refugees out of Saigon (this was in 1975, at the end of the Vietnam War), and he could barely speak any English, but he was a serious man who didn't waste any time. He walked into that room on the first day, ready to spar. Keith will never forget that first session. The teacher grabbed his hand, put it into a fist, and repeated the word. Fist, fist, fist, fist, fist.

That was his way of saying: Start with the basics. There are fifty thousand ways to make the wrong fist. Get the fist right first. Later, there would be spinning and kicking and all of that, but at first it was just fist, fist, fist. You cannot start with the complex and work back to the simple. That is a recipe for crashing and burning.

That's exactly how we advise people who ask us what they should eat. Fist, fist, fist. Simple, simple, simple.

So what's the simple version of the paleo diet? The paleo party line is essentially this: If you could dig it, pick it, or kill it with a spear, it was potential food. You could follow the program in any of dozens of books (we recommend anything by Mark Sisson, J. J. Virgin, Robb Wolf, Terry Wahls, Nora Gedgaudas, Pete Evans, Alan Christianson, or Chris Kresser, just to name a few of the many options out there). Or, you can do what Michelle recommends and start with the bare-bones basics for optimizing the human body and brain:

1. **Fresh vegetables** of all kinds, like leafy greens, broccoli, cauliflower, cabbage, asparagus, artichokes, squashes, and so on.
2. **Animal protein**—meat, poultry, seafood, and eggs.
3. **Roots and tubers**, like carrots, beets, potatoes, and yams.
4. **Nuts and seeds** of all types, raw or dry-roasted, and their butters (without additives). (Note that peanuts are legumes, not nuts.)

5. **Natural, minimally processed fats,** especially olive oil, avocado oil, coconut oil, cold-pressed nut oils, ghee (butter oil without whey solids), lard, and tallow.

6. **Optional: fresh fruit** if you need some extra love in your diet. It's part of the natural human diet, but it was typically only available during a limited time during the year, so early humans didn't eat it all the time.

Eat this way and you won't lack anything you need or get anything you don't need. This is paleo kindergarten: Just six simple things.

When we give people this dietary advice, we inevitably get a string of questions: What kind of meat? (Any kind.) How do I cook it? (Broil, grill, bake, or sauté, with coconut oil, ghee, olive oil, or avocado oil.) What counts as a root or tuber? (Anything that grows underground.) What if I don't want to eat meat? (Then don't.) If I take the patty off my Big Mac and throw away the bun, does that count? (Not ideal, but if you scrape off all the mystery sauce, it's animal protein.) What about French fries? (No, those are processed. Just eat a potato.)

Don't let the questions hold you back. Don't worry about being perfect. Don't torture yourself over the details. Don't concern yourself with

---

PETE EVANS SAYS . . .

As you look at the big picture of how and what you eat, it's also important to consider the "Bigs" picture. Our friend Pete Evans is an internationally renowned chef, restaurateur, entrepreneur, keynote speaker, author, television presenter, and documentary producer. Keith recently interviewed Pete on a podcast, and he said:

> If each and every one of us chose never again to purchase a food product made by a multinational food company, the trickle-down effect of that would change not only the world economy, but world governance overnight. We are that powerful as individuals and as a collective.

Amen, brother!

portion sizes. Just *start*. In the beginning, keep it simple simple simple. Try it for just two weeks and see how much better you feel. Then you can work on refining. Don't let the perfect get in the way of the good.

Once people get off all the processed food, they begin to see for the first time what's really in their kitchen cabinets and pantries: a bunch of crap. Michelle doesn't tell them to start by cleaning out their cabinets because people always resist. They don't want to throw away food. Once they start feeling the transformation happening, they suddenly see what they have been eating, and they get rid of it on their own.

After you get those six basics right, you can begin adding things to see how that feels, and improving the quality of your food. At first, we never

BEYOND PALEO KINDERGARTEN

Here's how to level-up your paleo:

1. **Better vegetables.** Look for organic and/or locally grown vegetables of all kinds. Try new veggies often. Variety provides the widest range of micronutrients and seasonal choices will be the most nutritious.
2. **Cleaner animal protein.** Ideally organic and preferably grass-fed, pastured, or wild-caught, animal protein has more options than you might think. Try game meats like bison, elk, ostrich, and venison. Seek out local farmers who sell directly. If you hunt or know a hunter, you could expand your animal protein repertoire even more. Experiment with different kinds of wild-caught seafood (stay away from farmed varieties).
3. **More nutritious roots and tubers.** Also ideally organically grown because they are in direct contact with the soil, roots and tubers will be more nutritious in richer soil. These are great sources of resistant starch and fiber for feeding your microbiome and encouraging microbial diversity, especially if you don't scrub them too vigorously. Traces of clean organic dirt are good for you.
4. **Soaked raw nuts and seeds.** Most nutritious when they are raw, soaking and drying nuts and seeds before eating can

reduce the lectin content. If you prefer them roasted, avoid industrial vegetable oils. To DIY your nuts and seeds, soak, dry, and roast them with avocado oil and sea salt.

5. **Quality fats.** Source them the way you would animal protein. Avoid industrially produced vegetable oils like canola, sunflower, safflower, soy, and that enigmatic "vegetable oil," and rancid olive oil. We prefer organic virgin coconut oil; lard, tallow, and ghee from grass-fed or pastured animals; and the highest quality olive oil, such as Kasandrinos (you can visit our online Resources page at PrimalUprising.com/BookResources for information on sourcing).

6. **Seasonal fruit.** Favor low-sugar, high-nutrient fruits like berries, but any fruit that is in season will be nutritious and fiber-packed. You may do better with just a little fruit, or you may do fine eating several servings a day. Notice how your body reacts to fruit. Fruit is a pleasure, but it's not necessary for good health.

Don't let any of this stress you out. Do the best you can with what you've got. If you can afford to pay for grass-fed meat and organic vegetables and fruits, fabulous. If not, at the end of the day, the most important thing is to get the processed food out. Make the best possible decisions, then be at peace. You're going to have success as long as you stick to the basics.

mention quality because if it sounds too complicated or expensive, people may not sustain it. Master the perfect fist first, then branch out where it makes sense to you.

As you work on these changes, you will probably crave processed food—especially foods that are sugary or salty/crunchy. These foods have been made cheap and hyperpalatable on purpose. Dallas Hartwig and Melissa Hartwig Urban, who wrote *It Starts with Food* and *Whole 30*, call these "food with no brakes" because they turn off your satiety receptors. Remember that potato chip commercial, "Bet you can't eat just one?" Those chips have been engineered that way.

In the last chapter, we told you about optimal foraging theory. These instincts that once saved our lives and insured the continuation of our species now threaten to do just the opposite. You're not always going to do everything in your own best interest. Welcome to life. If you can limit the "food with no brakes" to once-in-a-while and special occasions, you can still stay healthy.

What's Not on the List?

We aren't into the concept of "bad foods," but there are certain kinds of foods—namely most grains, legumes, dairy products, and sugar—that have not been part of the natural human diet for a reason. Before we began farming in earnest, humans really didn't eat much in the way of grains or legumes, due to naturally occurring toxins and more complex preparation requirements. Dairy was consumed in only very small parts of the world, mostly by nomadic herding tribes in northern Europe (people of northern European descent tend to be the only people who can easily digest dairy products). Refined sugar simply didn't exist.

People often argue that there is nothing wrong with grains, legumes, or dairy foods. For those who aren't sensitive, that may be true, but here's what we know about why you may choose to avoid them:

1. **Gluten** is a protein in wheat, rye, barley, spelt, and other grains that is hard for most people to digest and inflammatory for many, leading to the general paleo guideline to avoid gluten-containing grains. Some people extend this to include all grains, citing research that grains in general are inflammatory and not a significant part of the original human diet. Others make exceptions for small amounts of non-gluten-containing ancient grains like quinoa and wild rice (not technically grains), or organic and heirloom corn.

2. **Casein** (a protein in dairy products) and **lactose** (a sugar in dairy products) can be hard to digest and inflammatory, leading to a general guideline to avoid all dairy products. Some people make

exceptions for full-fat organic dairy products; dairy from goat milk or sheep milk; or, better yet, raw dairy products (which are unpasteurized and absurdly illegal in some states, even though the risks are minimal and people have been eating raw dairy products for thousands of years—visit our online Resources page at PrimalUprising.com/BookResources to find the laws in your state on raw milk).

There are also two types of casein: A1 and A2. Different breeds of cows produce milk with different types of casein. Most of the dairy cows in the US produce A1 milk, which tends to be more inflammatory and harder to digest, with larger protein molecules. A2 milk, more common in the milk from European cows and those from Australia and New Zealand, produce the smaller-molecule, more digestible A2 casein. A2 milk has finally come more into the public consciousness and is easier to find than it used to be. The one dairy exception Michelle allows is a splash of A2 full-fat creamer in her morning coffee. It doesn't upset her stomach the way A1 does.

3. Anti-nutrients like **lectins and phytates** are high in legumes and grains, and can block mineral absorption. Some people make exceptions for the most easily digested legumes like lentils, or soak legumes and nongluten grains until they sprout, to reduce lectin and phytate content. Pressure cooking also reduces these anti-nutrients.

There are more restrictive versions of the paleo diet, often designed for people with health conditions such as autoimmune diseases, that may limit other food categories such as nightshade vegetables (tomatoes, peppers, potatoes, eggplant, and goji berries) and eggs. There are also trendy (but valid) versions, such as the aforementioned Whole 30, keto (short for ketogenic), and carnivore diets. Whatever you choose, it's an opportunity for you to make your own food decisions, and ultimately move toward greater health and food freedom.

THE KETO CRAZE

Keto is having its 15 minutes of fame. A true ketogenic diet consists of a high level of fat—65 to 90 percent or more of calories from fat—which leaves very little room for carbs and protein, and most people "on keto" are probably eating less fat than that. The original purpose of the ketogenic diet was therapeutic. It was used for people with epilepsy or severe obesity because it seemed to help control seizures and caused rapid weight loss. The mechanism is to exhaust the body's glucose supply so that it has to switch to burning fat (technically, ketone bodies) for fuel. This state of fat burning is called ketosis. The theory is that this is more beneficial for the body and especially the brain, and that it's the fastest way to burn off body fat.

Typical keto foods include coconut oil or MCT (medium-chain tri-glyceride) oil, avocadoes, nuts and seeds and their butters, olive oil, meat, and non-starchy vegetables. Some also use eggs, and other animal fats like lard. Although dairy foods aren't classically a part of a paleo diet, some people on a ketogenic diet use full-fat dairy products like butter, cream, and ghee.

For most people who don't have a neurological disorder and are not severely obese, the ketogenic diet probably isn't necessary and may not be sustainable over the long term. For some, it can cause high cholesterol. Some argue that it can and should be a long-term diet because the body and brain benefits are worth the effort it takes to get and stay in ketosis. Others caution those with a family history of heart disease against this high-fat way of eating. There are many opinions on the subject, so if it interests you, we suggest you do some research.

To learn more, check out our Resources webpage at PrimalUprising.com/BookResources to find links to the Ketogains website and Keto Masterclass, and our own site, Keto f(x).

Food Sensitivities

Food sensitivities are highly individual. One person might be lactose intolerant, another might react to nightshade vegetables. Some people get digestive distress from almonds or mouth swelling from cantaloupe or joint pain after eating eggs. Just because a food is healthy for some doesn't mean it's good for *you*. You may already have an idea of what foods seem to bother you, just because you've noticed you get digestive pain, fatigue, or other uncomfortable symptoms after eating them. Or, you might not think you have a food sensitivity because you are so used to the pain and discomfort you experience regularly.

One way to find out if you have food sensitivities is to keep a journal of foods and symptoms so you can track patterns, but the best way to know what food sensitivities you have is to do an elimination test. To do this on your own, stick to a limited diet for a few weeks (such as the basic paleo diet Michelle recommends on page 57–58, then try introducing the suspected foods one at a time and pay attention to how your body reacts. You may find that as you get healthier, you are able to reintroduce small amounts of these foods once in a while, or you may feel best if you leave them out of your diet for good. Your body is a diagnostic tool—it is constantly giving you feedback. You just need to listen to it.

There are some tests that can determine whether you are having inflammatory or immune reactions to foods, like IgE (allergy), IgG, and IgA tests, but these don't always coincide with noticeable symptoms. They can still be useful, however: Sometimes you just need to see test results to push yourself to do what you already know you need to do. Some good testing companies include Everlywell, Cyrex, and Apeiron. Some tests require a doctor's prescription, but many don't. We think DIY lab tests will be increasingly accessible to all.

Thoughts on Animal Cruelty

There is a lot of unfortunate sniping between "paleo people" and "plant-based people," which is too bad, because the paleo and plant-based communities have more in common than they often realize. Both generally believe in a whole-food, natural diet, eating a lot of plant foods, and both have a beef (so to speak) with the Standard American Diet and especially the industrial food system. They differ on whether or not humans should eat meat, but they do not differ on their disgust with the unethical treatment of factory-farmed animals.

Our friends Diana Rodgers and Robb Wolf recently collaborated on a book and companion documentary, both called *Sacred Cow*, that argue for the inclusion of sustainably and ethically produced meat. Confined animal feeding operations are extremely environmentally destructive and produce the least healthy meat. Big Ag tells us this is necessary to feed the world, but millions of tons of food are wasted every year, while people continue to starve. Animals are treated as little profit systems (sound familiar?), not living beings. They are shot up with growth hormones and chemical antibiotics. They are often sick and killed while fearful.

We're going to get a little mystical here, but we believe everything that goes into an animal goes into you when you eat that animal. You are eating the hormones, chemicals, disease, and even the fear. You can taste that fear—it's gamy and strange. It may sound "woo" but you are tasting the adrenaline and cortisol in the animal killed while in a fight-or-flight stress state. We think that eating this cruelty and violence could play a role in the high rates of depression.

Every animal deserves a good life, frolicking in the pasture, chewing cud, pecking for insects, or doing whatever is natural for that animal to do. Nobody should have to live crammed into a battery cage stacked ten chickens high with chicken poop falling down through the cages. Nobody should have to live in a gestation crate, unable to move, or stuffed into a pen standing in their own waste. Nobody should have to live a life of suffering, fear, pain, disease, and untimely death. We can't imagine what human ever thought it was okay to treat animals like this.

It's up to us to demand something different. If most people saw how their food animals lived, they would probably never want to eat meat again, and we don't blame them. It's horrific, but people are so disconnected from their food and so traumatized by the idea of this level of cruelty that they push it deep into their subconscious and pretend it's not happening. But it's inside of you.

Let's let it out and demand change. When animals kill each other for food, it's natural, but it's also violent and vicious. We can do nature one better in this instance. We can give animals a death that is respectable and honors the life they lived. We can refuse to waste an animal, so nobody dies in vain. Then, we can give back. When we die, we go back to the earth and we feed the grass, insects, and animals, creating nutrients to grow grass and other plants that the animals can consume, and it all starts again. It's the rolling circle of life.

What About Supplements?

Keith once set out to prove he could eat a perfect diet from food alone without any supplementation, but he ended up proving the opposite. After going without supplements for six months, he did some nutrient testing and found he was deficient in omega-3 fatty acids and vitamins D and K, with suboptimal levels in a few other key areas. He realized he needed supplementation to get all the nutrients his body requires. He determined that he could theoretically get everything he needed if he lived in a pristine, unpolluted world with a rich soil microbiome full of minerals, and ate a wide variety of plant foods and organ meat. Unfortunately, that scenario is basically no longer possible without major changes to our world. That takes us to supplements.

Supplements can be confusing. Many supplements don't contain what they say they contain, and may also be adulterated with heavy metals or other toxins. We don't want to tell you what to do or take (we're not Big Paleo!) but we do like to share things that work for us, and one of those is the company IDLifeWellness, which offers customized supplement packs—they don't cut corners, and their supplements are pure and bio-available. We take them ourselves (and work with them, full disclosure). On their website, IDLifeWellness.com, you can take a free assessment to see what supplements you need. It's not the only high-quality brand—there are lots of great supplement companies. Look for supplements you have researched, with independently verified quality control. And as always, whether or not you take them is and always should be *your decision*.

SHAWN WELLS SAYS . . .

Our friend Shawn Wells is a product formulator and expert in performance nutrition. He's a supplement guru, and this is his advice on the basic supplements almost everyone should be taking:

The Standard American Diet (SAD) truly is sad and lacks many essential nutrients. To make up for this lack, I recommend taking these supplements:

> **Vitamin D3** is critical for the immune system and a hormone involved in mood, fat storage/obesity, insulin sensitivity, bone health, and more things we continue to find. I recommend 5,000 IU of D3 daily (or 10,000 IU during winter months in the northern half of the US). I also recommend taking vitamin D with vitamin **K2 - MK7** at a dose of 100 to 300 mcg once or twice daily, for best effects.

> **Magnesium** (my favorite form is glycinate, standardized to 120 mg of elemental magnesium twice per day) is responsible for more than two hundred enzymatic processes, including immunity, muscle contraction, focus/mood, sleep quality, bowel motility, and much more.

> **Methylcobalamin** and **5-MTHF** (the co-enzyme forms of vitamin B12 and folic acid, also known as active B12 and active folate) protect you neurologically. They are also involved in methylation (protecting DNA), give you energy, and reduce homocysteine levels. Take 1 to 5 mg of both methylcobalamin and 5-MTHF twice a day.

> **Creatine** is so much more than a bodybuilding compound. It creates creatine phosphate in the body that, yes, can improve power and strength, muscle recovery, and growth, but it also protects against DNA damage (as a methylator) and improves bone health, reproductive health, and eye health, and potently protects brain health. Take 2.5 to 5 grams per day.

> **Omega 3s** from fish oil in the triglyceride or phospholipid form, at a dosage of 2 to 3 grams of fish oil a day, will reduce systemic inflammation, improve cardiovascular

health, protect the brain, and improve triglycerides (a type of fat found in blood—too much can raise the risk of heart disease).

> **Berberine** (or the active dihydroberberine, which is even better) is an anti-glycation agent (meaning, it prevents the glycotoxins called advanced glycation end products or AGEs, which cause inflammation) that promotes glucose disposal. It's anti-inflammatory, improves blood sugar and insulin sensitivity, improves triglycerides, and is the ultimate ingredient I've found to promote longer life and reduce disease risk metabolically. I recommend 500 mg (or 150 mg of dihydroberberine) 3 times per day with meals.

> **Alpha-GPC** is the most bioavailable form of choline that can pass the blood-brain barrier, increasing acetylcholine (a neurotransmitter) levels and improving phospholipids in the brain. It has been shown in studies to improve sleep, strength and power, focus, and much more. I recommend 300 to 600 mg 3 times per day.

> **Ashwagandha**, **lion's mane**, and **rhodiola** are, collectively, a class of herbs known as adaptogens, which should be cycled as needed. I personally use one bottle of one of these, then move on to a bottle of the next one, and so on.
>   ► Look for ashwagandha with a higher anolide extract content, such as in Sensoril—I recommend 250 mg twice per day.
>   ► For lion's mane, look for 30 to 50 percent polysaccharides, including the active secondary metabolites hericenones and erinacines, 300 to 500 mg twice daily.
>   ► Rhodiola should have a high salidroside content like in RhodioPrime, dosage 400 to 600 mg twice per day. All of these adaptogens normalize numerous body functions, through optimization.

One can expect greater resilience and ability to manage stress and, with that, improved sleep, strength/power, immune system function, blood sugar control, mood, and much more.

In closing this chapter, we want to emphasize that we all have the same nutritional needs when it comes to broad strokes, but we are all also highly individual, so when it comes to the details, there is a range of what each person can eat to be healthy. When in doubt, just go back to those basic six: vegetables, meat, roots/tubers, nuts/seeds, healthy fats, and fruit. For most people, this is all that is necessary for feeling transformed. Then you can move on to the other six pillars of health.

PRIMAL UPRISING LITMUS TEST

> Am I actually hungry? Would an apple or a salmon salad satisfy me, or do I only want junk?
> What am I eating that my body doesn't need?
> Am I eating the basic six? Do I have a good reason to be eating anything else?

5

FREE TO MOVE

A human being should be able to change a diaper, plan an invasion, butcher a hog, conn a ship, design a building, write a sonnet, balance accounts, build a wall, set a bone, comfort the dying, take orders, give orders, cooperate, act alone, solve equations, analyze a new problem, pitch manure, program a computer, cook a tasty meal, fight efficiently, die gallantly. Specialization is for insects.

—Robert A. Heinlein, science fiction author

After improving your food, the next step to optimizing the human body is fitness. Imagine a soft, overweight, weak, frail, fatigued zoo animal trying to escape. To hone your fitness and maximize your energy is to train for your life as a free human. You can build an active, responsive, adaptable, strong, flexible body that is prepared for anything, whether crisis or opportunity. When your moment comes, will you be ready?

We believe the best way to train the human body is to look back to what our bodies needed to do for us before we lived in an easy, automated world. For all of our twenty-first-century tech advances, we are still walking around in bodies with an ancient design that evolved many millennia before humans ever sat at desks or on couches looking at screens. Our ancestors moved the way they had to move to survive, which made them versatile. They had to be able to run away, run after, walk far, jump over, crawl under, carry heavy things, push, pull, lift, throw, swim, and of course, rest and recover. Movement was essential for survival.

Today, we don't need to move all that much, so a lot of people today see exercise purely as a way to look better. That's great, but some people forget that exercise is the most important way for the human body to stay functional for years to come. If you exercise regularly and you have strength and endurance, life takes less effort. No matter what you are doing—hauling groceries, doing yard work, picking up toddlers, or just relaxing—muscle makes it easier.

Think of a human doing gymnastics, yoga, ice skating, skiing, swimming, surfing, diving, dancing, doing triathlons, climbing mountains, hang gliding. It's mind-boggling what humans have physically achieved. Something about us makes us want to push the envelope and do things nobody has ever done before. That's why people are always breaking records in sports and in pursuits like climbing the highest mountain or being the fastest to sail around the world.

ERWAN LE CORRE SAYS . . .

Our friend Erwan Le Corre is the founder of MovNat and author of *The Practice of Natural Movement*. These are his wise thoughts on human movement and how the mind can direct what the body can do:

Regardless of the particular physical activity you're into, the idea that physical training is only physical doesn't reflect reality. Think about it: Beyond the autonomic system, the body only performs the very movements and efforts you're ordering it to do. There's always an agenda that drives your own chosen physical expression and that intent doesn't stem from your muscles . . . muscles don't have a mind of their own. Whether you seek movement mastery, body aesthetics, physical capability, the inherent satisfaction of the activity itself, or all of the above, it starts with a pursuit born from your own mind, your own spirit.

But what an athlete does—specialize—is different from what humans have traditionally done, which is generalize. If you are not a professional athlete and you want to train your body for life in general, you will train to be a generalist. You don't want to be so muscle-bound that you can't run for a mile, but you don't want to be so trimmed down for running a marathon that you can't lift a fifty-pound bag of concrete off the ground.

You want to be able to do it all, just in case you have to. You want to be able to respond physically to unexpected situations. Life is full of surprises and you never know when you might need to be fit. Natural human movement is a gift humans are given at birth, and ideally they should be able to retain that gift all the way to the end of their lives.

CHRIS LORANG AND ABBIE SAWYER SAY . . .

Chiropractor Chris LoRang and his partner Abbie Sawyer are creators of and leaders in the very cool "baby-led movement" and the authors of the *Baby-Led Movement Guide*. Here's what they have to say about primal infant movement and how to prevent orthopedic problems in a baby's future:

> People don't often give much thought to how their babies learn to move, but when babies are allowed to take the lead in their own physical development, the benefits are remarkable and lifelong. We propose that a minimalistic evolutionary model for infant movement is superior to any device, and that parents and caregivers can intervene in a beneficial rather than detrimental way by avoiding all devices or assistance that hinder or alter natural movement. Unless a baby can get into a position or movement completely on their own—like sitting up or walking on two feet—they should not artificially experience this position through the aid of a device or assistance. When infants have free-range and baby-led movement, you can observe the innate and incredible process of a baby learning how to move. Baby-led movement provides the "nutrients" necessary to build the foundation of the human biomechanical system.

Assessing Your Fitness

When Keith assesses the fitness of someone seeking training, here are the basic tests he uses to determine physical functionality. You can do these for yourself at home:

1. **Can you lie on the ground, then stand up without holding onto anything, including the floor?** This is harder than it sounds— even some of Keith's younger clients can't do it. This is a test that researchers use to gauge general health and longevity.

2. **Can you sit in a squat with your feet flat?** This is a great indicator of flexibility as well as leg strength. This is how people often sat before they had chairs. Extra points if you can sit into a squat, then stand back up without using your hands.

3. **How long does it take you to walk (or run) a mile as fast as you can?** In general, a moderately fit man should be able to do this in nine minutes, and a moderately fit woman should be able to do it in a little over ten minutes, thirty seconds.

4. **How long can you hang from a bar without your feet touching the ground?** A moderately fit man should be able to do this for thirty seconds, and a moderately fit woman should be able to do this for twenty seconds.

If you ace these tests, congrats and keep going. If not, don't worry. One of our favorite sayings is: *No failure, only feedback.* How you perform on these tests is only a measure of where you are right now, not any indication of your limits. Even athletes can have trouble with these tests. One of Keith's clients, an accomplished cyclist, could ride a hundred miles at a blistering pace, but there was no way he could get up off the floor without using his hands. He was a specialist, but he wasn't adaptable. He was optimized only for cycling.

Consider this inspiration to achieve your next goal, or micro-goal, which might be to get off the floor using only one hand, walk a mile thirty seconds faster than the last time, or hang for five seconds longer. An inch of progress is an inch in the right direction. If you let regular exercise be your path to adaptability, you will see progress on these fitness tests, and you'll quickly begin to notice how much easier everyday life gets. (If you want to get more high-tech about it, check out realFIT, which gamifies fitness in a cool way, with various fitness tests and scores. Find the link in our Resources webpage at PrimalUprising.com/BookResources.)

YOUR GENETIC FITNESS

A genetic test can tell you many things about your propensities, vulnerabilities, susceptibilities, and strengths. One interesting thing you can learn is whether you have more muscle fibers that make you a better sprinter (fast-twitch muscle fibers) or better at endurance (slow-twitch muscle fibers). This can suggest what kind of sports you might be good at, although it's not destiny—you can train for anything. (Keith has the genetics of an endurance athlete, but he much prefers speed and power and detests "long and slow." Michelle has the genetics of an elite athlete, but competitive sports aren't all that interesting to her.)

Our favorite genetic testing companies are Apeiron, which is more comprehensive, and IDLifeWellness DNA tests, which are more specific to fitness and nutrition. For links, visit our Resources webpage at PrimalUprising.com/BookResources.

Your Metabolic Currency

Muscle is metabolic currency, and if exercise were a pill, it would be the most potent cure on the market today, especially for diabetes. Muscle burns blood sugar, utilizes fat, increases bone density, releases human growth hormone to combat aging, and makes us less likely to fall—and less likely to get injured if we do.

The way to build muscle is through load-bearing, but the method and the weight involved varies according to the individual. To an eighty-year-old woman who has never exercised, walking around the block would be load-bearing. To a guy like Keith who has been lifting weights since he was twelve years old, load-bearing means he has to hoist some heavy-ass weights. Only you can know what level of load-bearing will challenge you and push you just outside your comfort zone without being too easy or causing injury. Don't worry about looking muscle-bound. At thirty minutes twice a week, you won't be Mr. or Ms. Olympia, but you will be strong and adaptable.

FOR THOSE WITH PHYSICAL LIMITATIONS

Having physical limitations is no reason not to keep moving. Do what you can, move what you can, and do it every day. You never know what you can accomplish until you try. Those with limitations have accomplished great feats of athletic prowess. Let them be your inspiration and move something, anything, as often as you can. As Kyle Manard (a quadruple amputee athlete who climbed Mount Kilimanjaro without prosthetics and is the author of *No Excuses*) says, "Know your limits, but never stop trying to break them." If you aren't sure what to do, a trainer or physical therapist can help you design a plan that works with what you *can* do.

If you spend most of your day sitting (as most people do), you are probably thinking that you could use a little more movement in your life. Sitting is part of a digital world, but we don't have to be captive to a screen (consider a standing desk—Keith also stands on a wobble board to raise the stakes). All exercise makes a difference, but strength does more for you than anything else. Here's what a physically adaptable human should be able to do:

Walk: This is the most basic human movement. Our ancestors had to walk to get water, forage, hunt, and follow the herds. Walking won't get you into superior cardiovascular condition, but it's one of the most useful life skills and humans have always had to do it (we hope they always will). If you aren't doing any exercise at all right now, walking is the place to start, especially over uneven or undulating terrain. Maybe brush up on your cycling skills, too. We believe that a physically versatile human should be able to walk (or the equivalent) for at least a mile, ride a bike for at least a couple of miles, and climb a few flights of stairs without feeling like they are going to keel over. Hey, if it all goes down someday and all the fuel runs out and we have to go back to a more primitive form of living, you're going to be glad you can get around on your own steam.

Sprint: While there were tribes that ran long distances, most of our ancestors, when they did have to run, had to do it fast and for short bursts. Those who survived were the best sprinters, and we descended from them, so it's something most can potentially do (even if some people do it better—we're looking at you, Usain Bolt). Luckily for us, sprinting doesn't have to come with a tiger on your heels or a gold medal on the line. We can sprint for fun, rather than for our immediate survival. Sprinting is a key element of metabolic health and physical fitness. Start by adding short sprints to your daily walk or jog. Every five minutes or so, break into a short sprint, as hard and fast as you can. Start with five for twenty seconds and work up to a couple of minutes. This is a great way to build your cardiovascular fitness fast, and if you ever really do need to run to save your life, you'll have the capacity to do it.

Push, pull, hinge, squat, carry, drag, and swing: Weight-bearing doesn't have to mean sweating it out in a gym (although it could). What matters is that you can lift heavy things, hold them above your head, push them, pull them. Think about all the things a hunter-gatherer had to do to survive: carry the deer, elk, or bison back to camp; haul water and forage for food; build shelters and carry firewood; roll stones and logs; hoist an ax; pull a cart; and a million other physical things. You may not have to carry heavy things most of the time, but what if you had to carry someone out of a burning building or rescue someone drowning in a lake? Add these movements to your survival arsenal.

ANDY GALPIN SAYS . . .

Andy Galpin is a professor of muscle physiology and human performance at Cal State Fullerton and the author of *Unplugged*. He and Keith concur on prioritizing muscle strength. Here are his thoughts:

> Nothing is more central to both lifespan and wellness than muscle. It not only controls physical movement but also regulates countless physiological processes critical to human function. The quality and depth of science behind this is astounding and beyond reproach. Muscle also has a robust ability to fix problems in other areas. Muscle isn't the only thing important to health, but it's probably the biggest.

The bottom line is adaptability. There is no preset sequence of activities that works for everyone or that will build total fitness. Switch it up and find ways to use multiple types of movements at once. For instance, this morning Keith did handstand push-ups. He was lifting his own body weight, pushing away from the floor, and balancing. It's weight-bearing but it also gets his heart rate up, it's proprioceptive so it improves cognitive function—it's a kind of mental jujitsu—and it's both gymnastic and fun. You don't need to divide and categorize your workout. You can flow in and out of cardio, weight-bearing, and athletics. We see exercise as a big circle of different kinds of movements that can be combined into flow-type activities as well as locomotion. For example, when Keith travels, he'll head out into the city and walk for three minutes, do lunges for a minute, then do forty push-ups. Is it weight-bearing? Locomotion? Flow? Yes. To Keith, this is interesting and fun, no matter how strange it might look to pass-ersby. We envision natural human movement something like this:

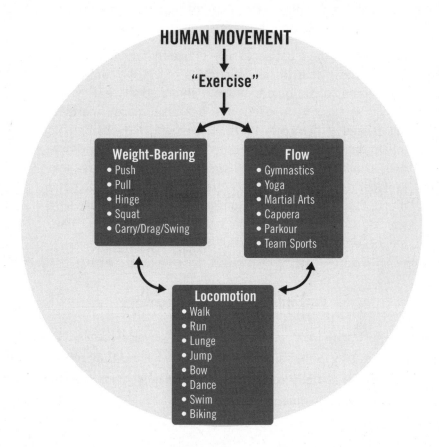

Jump on this wheel at any point and take a ride. When you've had enough, jump off. You never need to feel limited to any one category, or feel like you need to do exercise X for Y minutes, Z times a week. Just move. Push yourself. Experiment with what your body can do, and how it changes as you get fitter and stronger. Have fun. Play. Get inspired by movement you see out there in the world, and use your creativity. You know how to do this.

DARRYL EDWARDS SAYS . . .

Our friend Darryl Edwards, who teaches a fun kind of movement called Primal Play, is an expert at finding ways to play in urban settings. He's the publisher of PrimalPlay.com and the best-selling author of *Animal Moves*. Here's what he says about human movement:

> Movement is the most accessible of health interventions. It's free and available for all, regardless of age or ability, and it's one critical antidote to modern chronic disease. Physical activity is proven to reduce the risk of all-cause mortality (all causes of death) by up to 50 percent, reduces chronic inflammation, and reduces the risk of metabolic syndrome and insulin resistance. Movement can also improve lipid profiles, reduce cancer risk, enhance cognitive function and mood, too. Above all, it just makes us feel better. Make sure you are taking your movement prescription daily and have lots of fun to get even more out of it!

Flexibility, Rest, and Recovery

Balance effort with recovery for maximum physical fitness. Flexibility helps the body stay limber and resilient. People believe they get stiffer with age, but stiffness actually comes from lack of movement over time. Rest gives your body the chance to repair micro-damage to muscles, making them stronger. For maximum recovery, get seven to nine hours of sleep a night and eat enough protein. (Keith generally recommends 1 gram of protein per pound of lean bodyweight. Calculate your lean bodyweight with the US Navy Body Fat Calculator. Find it on our online Resources page at PrimalUprising.com/BookResources.)

FITNESS BIOHACKS

Biohacking, or using technology and other means to track and tweak the human body and human health, is big in the fitness world. Some of the more common biohacking tech includes fitness trackers that tell you how many steps you took, how many calories you burned, what your heart rate was, and so on, as well as sleep trackers, pulse-ox trackers, stress trackers, blood glucose monitors, and so much more. It seems like new products and technology come out every day. We think that what the biohacking community is doing is important because it brings awareness and knowledge.

However, although we both have smart watches, we don't go overboard with fitness tracking. It's too easy to get obsessive about it, and it can start to feel like you yourself are just a data point. We keep track of the basics—for instance, Michelle always tries to get in ten thousand steps a day—but for the most part, we keep our movement more natural, intuitive, and inspired by our hunter-gatherer forebears. However, if the trackers and hacks are useful for you and motivate you, then by all means, check them out. You can find a list of some of our favorite companies making cool biohacking tech at our online Resources webpage (PrimalUprising.com/BookResources), but remember that these devices are just tools to help you relearn how to listen to your body. Don't let the tool become a shackle.

The Best Exercise

What's the best exercise of all? The one you will actually do consistently. You know best what works for you. Keith was a football player and he loves team sports, but we know many people would much rather put on their headphones and exercise without any interaction. Some want to exercise only outside in nature; for others, the gym is bliss. Yoga isn't our thing; but for some people, it's the best exercise bar none and we have seen some pretty ripped yoga teachers.

Find your own natural way to move, and do something every day—at least thirty minutes, or up to ninety minutes of continuous movement, will change your life if you aren't doing it now. Really, the only thing that is totally unnatural for the human body is to sit at a desk staring at a computer all day, then lie on a couch staring at a television all night. Anything else is fair game. You don't have to make rules for yourself. Just move.

Maybe you have only twenty minutes to get in a workout today. That's twenty minutes longer than nothing. There are *many* days when twenty minutes is all any of us have. Just do something, and mix it up whenever you can. Remember the importance of staying physically adaptable.

PRIMAL UPRISING LITMUS TEST

> Do I move as much as I could?
> Can I lie down on the floor, then get up without using my hands?
> Can I sit in a squat position with my feet flat?
> How long does it take me to walk or run a mile?
> How long can I hang from a bar?
> Can I walk, sprint, and lift heavy things?
> Do I allow my body to recover?
> If I answered no to any of the above questions, what can I do to change my answer?

6

BECOMING PHYSICALLY RESILIENT

We do not rise to the level of our expectations. We fall to the level of our training.

—Archilochus

The last aspect of the physical pillar is resilience. Physical resilience is the ability of the body to adapt to any condition. If you are physically resilient, you could be dropped into the Arctic Circle or onto the equator and although it would be rough at first, you would survive in that new environment. This would eventually increase your resilience because stressing the body is what strengthens the body (like that repair that happens to muscles after weightlifting). It's true that what doesn't kill you makes you stronger. Stress combats fragility and builds resilience, and variable stress builds adaptability.

This is why athletes cross-train. They keep surprising their bodies with new movements and challenges so they never fall into a rut and get used to what they are doing. The human body is probably so good at adapting because throughout human history, those who were adaptable were the ones who survived. We may be at that point again. The modern world is full of challenges. It's time to adapt.

MICKRA HAMILTON SAYS . . .

Mickra Hamilton is the cofounder and CEO of the Apeiron Center for Human Potential/Apeiron Academy and a human performance subject matter expert in the US Air Force Reserves. She works on the cutting edge of human optimization and she says we are ready to evolve!

It is time to activate Precision Evolution, with the goal of purposefully evolving beyond our current narrow frame of resilience. It is no longer enough to bounce back from life stressors because our state of being is already diminished and depleted. We must cultivate an antifragile state, which places us in control of being better than we ever thought possible after encountering a hijack that comes down the evolutionary pike.

Can You Weather Any Storm?

When Keith was in the Navy at the end of the Cold War, he spent a lot of time in the North Atlantic where the oil fields are. Because of intel that Russia or one of its satellite nations might attack those oil fields (at the time, they provided the bulk of the oil for the US and Europe), the Navy patrolled that area. The North Atlantic is notorious for having storm after storm. The environment is punishing and the cold is bone-chilling. There were many times Keith thought they would all die out there.

But Keith is with us today, largely because of how those naval ships are built both offensively and defensively. If something goes wrong, no matter where it is, there is always a backup system ready to take over, so those ships are very hard to take down. Sinking a naval ship would require failure of the primary systems and all the backup systems before there was time to make repairs—so it rarely happens. The ships have been tested and tried by engineers who thought of all the possible ways the ships could fail. Naval ships are tough and built to withstand harsh conditions. They are resilient.

The human body is built a lot like those naval ships. It is tough and adaptable, and when something goes wrong, there are backup systems in place. The body is good at compensating, so if it takes a few hits from harsh conditions or incoming (metaphorical) fire, bam, your body can seal off that part of the ship and just keep on rolling. Maybe there's another hit, bam, and another hit, bam, and just as your body repairs one issue, you get another hit, bam. You can survive these storms for a while, and when the storm is over, you can make repairs. You may not thrive, but you can get by. But with more and more pings and hits and storms and no respite, eventually all those compensation systems *will* get worn down, your reserve will get used up, and then your ship is going to sink, like a beleaguered naval vessel. You're going to get sick. Your immune system, your detoxification system, your nervous system, your musculoskeletal system, your digestive system, your cardiovascular system . . . they can take a lot, but there is a limit.

You may not be able to control all your sources of stress, or the weather, pollution, the presence of viruses in the environment, or your genetic vulnerabilities, but you *can* control a lot, and you can make decisions based on how ship-shape you are at any given moment. When you're strong and resilient, you can take more stress, like heavy exercise, no sleep, a couple of cocktails, or some junk food. When you're already under a lot of stress, you might not fare so well taking those hits.

Whenever we make a decision about eating something that isn't what we would normally eat or doing something we know isn't great for us but we also know we will enjoy it, we ask ourselves, "Can I afford a hit to my battleship right now?" We consider how much sleep we've been getting, how regularly we've been exercising, how we've been eating, and how much stress we're currently enduring. Sometimes you want to take that hit, to combat fragility and increase resilience. Sometimes you don't because you're already in a weakened state. We are meant for stress. To quote author John A. Shedd, "A ship in harbor is safe, but that's not what ships are built for." But we're not *always* meant for stress.

Long before the COVID-19 pandemic, we were with friends who had traveled from every corner of the globe, as far-flung as China. We had just returned from international travel ourselves, and we all decided to have a party, even though we were tired and jet-lagged. Michelle knew she had to rest up, so she didn't drink any alcohol and she turned in early. Keith, on the other hand, stayed up all night partying and drinking beer, then swimming in the Pacific Ocean when the water felt like it was about 50 degrees. Cold exposure is a biohacking technique meant to improve physical resilience, but we weren't physically in a condition to handle it that night.

One of the women at the party had a cough, and within a couple of days, everyone who had stayed up late partying was brought to their knees by whatever respiratory virus she had. These were super-healthy people—biohackers and others in health-related fields who take really good care of themselves 99 percent of the time. This was one rare instance when we pushed ourselves past the point our resilience could handle. Keith was out of commission for a week, but not Michelle. She felt fine. Because she compensated for the jet lag and stress, her immune system was able to keep her from getting sick. Michelle found the whole thing hilarious. She called it our #biohackingfail. She was right. It was a fun night, but we paid dearly for it.

Becoming Hard to Kill

Right now, we don't live in a physically resilient population. Millennials are the first generation in modern times to be weaker and sicker and have shorter lifespans than their parents. Part of the problem is a stressful, polluted world, but another part is that we have it too easy. We live most of our lives indoors, and rarely expose ourselves to temperatures beyond an approximately 10- to 20-degree temperature range on either side of 70 degrees. We don't often exert ourselves except when we work out; most of us have never had to physically fight to survive. We eat the same favorite foods again and again, which can result in nutrient deficiency. When misfortune does suddenly visit, we are caught without reserves. Our battleships are rarely tested, so they aren't resilient.

What does it look like to be hard to kill? Here are some goals that can turn you into a physically resilient *thriver*:

- A normal body weight. This means a body mass index (BMI) generally between 18 and 25 or, better yet, an age/gender-appropriate body fat score, as measured by DEXA or Bod Pod. (See our Resources webpage at PrimalUprising.com/BookResources.)
- No nutritional deficiencies. A basic nutritional panel lab test can determine whether you are low in any vital nutrients, such as vitamin D, vitamin B12, or zinc.
- Smooth, easy digestion without cramping, bloating, constipation, or diarrhea.
- No chronic pain.
- Feeling physically healthy and strong.
- Illnesses and injuries that resolve or heal quickly.
- Healthy blood sugar balance with no pre-diabetes or diabetes.
- Good muscle tone and supple, flexible joints; a strong musculoskeletal system that can do whatever you need it to do.
- An intact gut lining—no "leaky gut syndrome," with food proteins leaking into the bloodstream, causing inflammation and immune reactions.
- A functional detoxification system with healthy liver and kidney function.
- A sharp, clear mind good at perceiving, learning, and problem-solving that can quickly, intelligently, and creatively respond to any situation.

To get ourselves resilient takes some purposeful cross-training of all these systems. Challenge your physical body and you send a message that it needs to get stronger. This is called hormetics, and it builds resilience. Our friend Charlie Deist, health advocate, radio producer, and the author of *Hormetics: Physical Fitness for Free People*, explains it this way: "Hormetics is the art of optimally applied beneficial stress." Here are some ways to use hormetics to build your resilience (when you're not overly stressed), so you can be hard to kill:

Change temperatures. Expose yourself to short bursts of extreme cold and high heat. You might be surprised how quickly and easily your body adjusts to life beyond 70 degrees. Some ways to do this include:

- Sitting in a sauna, then jumping in a cold pool.

- Standing outside on a very cold day, then taking a warm bath.

- Ending your daily shower with a minute or two of cold water.

- Waiting to turn on the air conditioner or the furnace in your home during the change of seasons for as long as you can.

Change elevation (or just hold your breath). If your body is exposed to different levels of oxygen, it will learn to adjust. Spend some time at high elevations when you can, but you can get similar benefits by practicing holding your breath. Start by holding it for just ten or twenty seconds a few times a day, then gradually work up to a minute or more.

Diversify your microbiome. The more "civilized" we get, the less diverse our microbiomes have become. These are the communities of microbes that live inside of us, mostly in our digestive tract. They assist with digestion, immunity, mood, stress management, and hormonal balance. Microbiomes are more robust and protect us better when they are more diverse (contain more species). Research has demonstrated that switching to a modern version of the Paleolithic diet, with a wide range of vegetables, meats, poultry, fish, nuts, seeds, and fruits, and also eating more seasonally, makes the human microbiome more diverse and more like those of modern hunter-gatherers.[12]

Switch from carb to fat burning. Spend a few weeks to a few months (or winter) in ketosis by eating very low-carb and high-fat, then switch to more carb burning for a few weeks to a few months (or in summer). Humans were naturally in ketosis more often in winter when plant foods were less available, and more likely burned glucose for fuel in summer when vegetables and fruits were at their peak of ripeness and sweetness. You can also achieve this effect through intermittent fasting.

LUIS VILLASEÑOR SAYS . . .

Our good friend Luis Villaseñor is a nutritionist and the founder of Ketogains, a keto protocol he developed to help achieve optimal body composition and health. Here's what he says about the benefits of ketosis:

> I started experimenting with ketogenic diets back in the winter of 1999, not really with the purpose of losing weight, as most people do, but to help me overcome anorexia and binge eating, and to gain lean muscle mass. I found out that eating whole, unprocessed foods made it incredibly easy for me to endure cravings and stay on the diet, while also improving my health exponentially. Over time, this experiment with keto became an actual coaching business. With the change of habits made possible by this way of eating, our clients were gaining lean mass, regaining health, and maintaining it for years.

Try intermittent fasting. Intermittent fasting is a less extreme form of fasting that's become trendy, but it's actually the way humans always used to eat. We all naturally fast while sleeping, but intermittent fasting extends this time to at least twelve hours (finishing dinner by 7:00 p.m. and not eating until 7:00 a.m., for example). Many people go longer: fourteen, sixteen, or eighteen hours. Some people practice the OMAD ("one meal a day") method of intermittent fasting. Intermittent fasting gives your digestion a break so your body can divert energy to other things like healing and detoxification, and promotes autophagy, which is the healthy removal of dead cellular matter from the body. If you haven't tried it before, start with twelve hours and work your way up from there, but also listen to your body's cues and don't fast longer than feels good to you.

DAVE ASPREY SAYS . . .

Our good friend Dave Asprey is the *New York Times* bestselling author of *Fast This Way* and CEO and founder of Bulletproof 360. Here are his latest thoughts on fasting:

Fasting isn't supposed to be scary. Intermittent fasting and longer fasts have always been a part of the human experience, except maybe the last one hundred years or so. We need fasting as a signal to make our cells more resilient. When we started working in factories, we swapped fasting for "three squares a day," which was great for Big Food manufacturers, but bad for your health. There is ample scientific evidence showing that various periods of fasting (that can be personalized, pin-pointed, and the results magnified—if you know a few tricks) are a boon to your overall physical health and vitality, not to mention your brain. It's the "biohack" that costs you absolutely nothing and pays immediate return in added time to your day. The physical and cognitive benefits? The best compound rate of return you'll ever get on an investment. When you know how to do it, you don't even feel hungry!

Break your exercise and work ruts. Shake up your exercise routine at least once or twice a week by doing some kind of exercise or movement totally different from what you usually do. Also be sure to include at least one day to rest and recover each week. That can mean stress-reducing activity like yoga, getting a massage, or just sleeping more.

Get dirty. Your immune system will become more intelligent if it is exposed to pathogens like viruses and bacteria, so don't be such a neat freak that you never touch dirt, get a scrape, or catch a cold, and don't overuse hand sanitizer. Keep it for when you really need it. (Especially avoid brands that contain deadly methanol![13]) Exposure to germs is what triggers your immune system to protect you. You should never

THE POMODORO TECHNIQUE

To shake up your work rut and sit less, try the Pomodoro technique: Work in short, intense bursts of twenty-five minutes (no peeking at social media), followed by a five-minute break with no work (no checking for that email from your boss), during which you get up and move around (vigorously if possible). This is one Pomodoro. After four Pomodoros, take a twenty-five-minute break to get up and move more, then start again. A total of twelve Pomodoros with their breaks is about equal to a full workday, and you won't get to the end of the day having been in a chair for eight hours straight. Many people swear by this routine and say it is a much healthier and more productive way to work.

Keith will sometimes vary this technique by alternating 90- to 120-minute work sessions with short breaks during which he does sixty kettle bell swings and drinks a glass of water. It's not really a workout, but it greatly increases his efficiency and he can work a twelve-hour day doing this.

put yourself into harm's way, of course, and your exposures should be measured and sensible, but research shows that people (especially kids) who are clean all the time and never play outside, touch animals, and put their hands and feet directly on the ground are more likely to have allergies and asthma.[14]

Free your liver. To keep your body's natural detoxification system operating at peak capacity and efficiency, free your liver to process what might come along, rather than keeping it constantly busy with incoming alcohol, junk food, and over-the-counter medications you take at the first sign of any discomfort. Instead, try herbal remedies and lifestyle changes like eating organic whole foods, moving more, sleeping more, and managing your stress, so your lymphatic system and liver are fresh and ready to handle the inevitable pollutants that we are all exposed to in the modern world.

DR. GUILLERMO RUIZ SAYS . . .

Our good friend Guillermo Ruiz, NMD, is a naturopath and an expert on endocrine disorders and botanical medicine. Here, he shares a few of his favorite, easily accessible herbal remedies:

I have spent years studying the healing power of plants and when I started applying ancestral wisdom to my experiments, things began to click. For centuries, many cultures have used plants as medicine, from Chinese Medicine to treat thyroid disease by using iodine rich algae to the native tribes of the southwest using plants as antibiotics. We have learned from trial and error how to take advantage of the gifts plants give us. Take for example the coffee plant. Through evolutionary adaptations, it created a little compound called caffeine to fight off insects. Caffeine is a naturally occurring insecticide that protects the plant. It just so happens that caffeine also increases focus and alertness in humans. Some of my favorite gifts from plants:

Ginger Tea: Ginger is a good treatment for post-operative nausea, and it also appears to help with motion sickness. *The Lancet* published a study in which participants were subjected to a nausea-producing apparatus. Those given the placebo lasted on the apparatus for 2.5 minutes and those who took Dramamine lasted 4.5 minutes. However, the participants who were given ginger lasted a full 6 minutes! Even better, ginger does not have drowsiness side effects like Dramamine. Researchers used powdered ginger in hot water, but ginger tea likely has the same or similar effect.

Echinacea Purpurea: The common cold is often caused by the rhinovirus, the most common pathogen associated with upper respiratory infections. Unfortunately, conventional medicine currently has no safe, approved treatment for these types of infections, but *Echinacea* has a long history of use as an immune modulator and antiviral. In double-blind placebo-controlled trials, it has been effective both as a prophylactic and in reducing the duration of symptoms. In a study by Sperber and friends, a group of healthy individuals was infected with rhinovirus and recorded symptoms and their duration. The patients treated with *Echinacea* experienced faster recovery.

Coffee and Honey: Coffee and honey have a long history of use as both food and medicine. Coffee is an antioxidant, expectorant, and hypoalgesic (decreases sensitivity to pain) while honey has been used for millennia to treat wounds and infections. Together, this power pair makes a tasty home remedy for that annoying cough that lingers after you've been sick. In fact, the synergy in this combination makes it more efficacious than oral steroids! Research on this natural cocktail demonstrates that it can completely resolve symptoms in a week.

Work hard, play hard. Alternate periods of hard work with periods of fun and relaxation. This will not only be good for mental resilience (see chapter 8), but it will help with your hormonal balance by regulating the output of stress hormones like cortisol and epinephrine.

Cleaning Up Your Environment

Constant exposure to toxins wears down the physical body and, over time, can drastically reduce physical resilience. We just aren't meant to live in a world teeming with environmental pollution, food chemicals, and sealed-up homes filled with artificial materials that off-gas and pollute our indoor air quality.

Living indoors with electricity and running water is pretty awesome, but you can reduce your toxic load and live more naturally. Some obvious steps are to use cleaning products and personal care products with natural ingredients, but here are some other ideas:

- **Go outside** at least a few times a day, even if you can only step outside your front door and breathe fresh air for a few minutes. Better yet, take daily walks or runs outside, or do your work sitting outside. Many studies have demonstrated that people who spend more time in nature are healthier and have more intelligent immune systems and more diverse microbiomes.

- **Open your windows** as often as possible. Not only will this improve your indoor air quality, but it will put you in closer contact with nature, as you feel the breeze, hear the sounds of birds or trees rustling, smell flowers or fresh-cut grass, and see green plants and blue sky.

- **Use natural materials** in your home as much as possible. Whenever you need to replace something, look for the most natural product you can. That can mean cleaning products and personal hygiene products, but it can also mean wood or bamboo flooring, rugs made from natural materials like wool and organic cotton, low-VOC paint, hardwood or metal furniture, stone or steel countertops, stainless steel pots and pans, and curtains and especially bedding made from natural materials. More natural products means less off-gassing.

- **Install water filtration and use air purifiers** to keep your water and air as clean as possible. We use a Santevia water filter and an Airocide air purifier. (Find links to these and other resources at PrimalUprising.com/BookResources.)

- **Bring the natural world inside** with plants, crystals, fountains, a (well-vented) fireplace or woodstove, and, if you are able to take care of them, pets. We also love the idea of natural-scaped yards with native plants instead of the old-school lawn concept that often requires dousing your property with chemicals to keep the lawn looking "respectable."

What the physical pillar really comes down to is optimizing an ancient body for life in a modern world. Work on this until you are feeling stronger, more capable, and more resilient. When you get your food and movement right and you begin to understand what it feels like to be so strong and capable, you'll get better at adapting to anything that comes at you. Next up, it's time to confront what's really going on inside your head.

PRIMAL UPRISING LITMUS TEST

> Do you occasionally expose yourself to extreme temperatures and/ or elevations?
> Have you tried intermittent fasting?
> Do you switch up your routine?
> How can you make your living environment less toxic and more natural?

PART III
THE
MENTAL
PILLAR

No man was ever wise by chance.

—Seneca the Younger

7

FREE TO THINK

It is the customary fate of new truths to begin as heresies.

—T. H. Huxley

You are destined to use your healthy and brilliant brain to think, question, consider, and be discerning. We live in a world where we cannot automatically assume what we hear is true—more than likely, when it comes to the powers that be, it's less true than a manipulation of truth meant to convince and control, divide and conquer. We are constantly exposed to aggressive efforts to shape our thinking, and we are not actively taught in our institutions of learning to think critically. We are taught *what* to think, not *how* to think, and that makes all the difference.

This is one of the primary ways we are kept in captivity. The bars of the cages of the human zoo are made out of manufactured or strategically selected but incomplete information meant to keep us inside the prison of our own small minds and limited beliefs. But you can have a big mind—an expansive, clear, rational, discerning mind. This isn't just desirable—it is necessary if you hope to ever be a truly free person. To be discerning is to remain skeptical, to question, and to wait to decide until you have enough information. We often don't have enough information, which means facing what we don't know and not jumping to conclusions based on knee-jerk, manipulated reactions. It's uncomfortable not to have a firm footing, but to be truly discerning is to get used to that discomfort.

PRIMAL WISDOM

The test of a first rate intelligence is the ability to
hold two opposed ideas in the mind at the same
time, and still retain the ability to function.
—F. SCOTT FITZGERALD

Getting Comfortable with Discomfort

We have a friend who is highly educated—she has a PhD—but she freely admits that she doesn't want to know the truth about what's really going on in the world. For her, ignorance is bliss. She's aware that something *is* going on "behind the curtain," but she values her bliss over the unease of knowing more. She just wants to live her life, she tells us, and whatever happens, happens. She has ceded control and allowed her mind to accept the mainstream narrative without question. That is her right, of course, but to us, she is the perfect example of someone who is book-smart but not discerning.

We are all free to think, but not everyone *chooses* to think. When we outsource our thoughts, we never achieve mental optimization and, by extension, mental freedom.

Will you accept whatever they tell you and stay under their control, or will you question and refuse to be duped? Do you respond or react? There are a lot of people out there preaching to their respective choirs right now, and the noise is a siren song. To be discerning is to be less concerned with being right and more concerned with constantly hunting for what is true.

If this feels intimidating or you feel unprepared to hurl yourself off the cliff of comfort, know that you can start small. The first step is just to question—not to blindly believe everything you hear, even if you are hearing what you want to believe is true or what makes you comfortable. When you think you know something, investigate it. Otherwise, it's all too easy to believe what you want to believe. When you start to feel just a little more skeptical of the messages you receive from out there in the world (including in this book), you are honing your own discernment. You are increasing your mental capacity for independent thought. Challenge authority. Defy dogma. Demand different.

How to Hone Your Discernment

How easy it is not to think. If we forget something, we can google it. If we don't know how to get somewhere, we can use the GPS. We don't need to know how to spell anymore and our kids aren't even taught cursive writing in school. Pretty soon, we won't have to drive our own cars. (The plump, junk food–bingeing, oblivious floating chair–bound humans in the movie *WALL-E* come to mind.)

The problem goes deeper. We no longer have to engage in civil discourse, hidden as we are by the filters and protection of digital communication. We don't have to be all that smart to be good enough. Becoming an expert is hard. Why bother? Who cares what's true when you can focus on what's amusing? Many people no longer understand the difference between facts and opinions, and don't get us started on what's happened to journalism, history, and the degradation of information. (Admittedly, we already did get started on some of that back in chapter 2.)

But you don't have to be mentally lazy. You can choose to hone your discernment and use your brain for your own benefit, rather than letting others use it for theirs. One way to do this is to force yourself to consider multiple viewpoints. On a daily basis, we expose ourselves to opinions that are opposite to our own, so while we admit to our biases, we are also aware of them and constantly questioning them.

We enjoy reading and listening to things we agree with, but we give equal time to those things that we know we will have a knee-jerk reaction against, and we constantly ask ourselves: "Is what we believe true?" "Is what they are saying true, even if we don't like it?" Keith keeps a Twitter list called "Love Thy Enemy," where he purposefully seeks out legitimate information outlets and knowledgeable people with points of view that are 180 degrees from his. He considers it his daily dose of castor oil.

THEO WILSON SAYS . . .

Our friend Theo Wilson has an unmissable TEDx talk about purposefully exposing oneself to opposing points of view, called "A Black
Man Goes Undercover in the alt-Alt-Right." Here are some of his
words from that talk:

America seems to be hell-bent on filling its textbooks with
CliffsNotes versions of its dark past. This severely decontex-
tualizes race and the anger associated with it. And that is
fertile ground for alt facts to grow.

This is how we guard against complacency. It's gymnastics for the
mind. What's more "true": a Breitbart article or an opinion piece from the
New York Times? The truth is probably somewhere in the middle. (You
don't agree? Question us, and question your immediate reaction to this
statement, too.) Sometimes the most provocative opinions can yield the
most food for thought.

Another thing we do is read more and keep the TV off. We and many of
our friends have stopped watching the news because Big Media has turned
the news into entertainment disguised as journalism. It spoon-feeds opinions to the masses rather than relaying a simple and unbiased version of
what happened. Those of us who've reached a certain vintage remember

HOW TO BE AN EPISTEMOCRAT

Keith has a blog called *Theory to Practice*, where he wrote a post
about being an epistemocrat. (Special thanks to our good amigo
Brent Pottenger and his fine blog Healthcare Epistemocrat, which
inspired Keith's blog post.) We thought it was appropriate to revisit
that post here, in an abbreviated form (check out Keith's blog to read
the entire post at PrimalUprising.com/BookResources).

An epistemocrat is a person who, concerned with what he or she does not know, engages in lifelong learning to embrace uncertainty. Essentially, an epistemocrat is a practitioner (a thinker and a doer) who respects the humble limits of being human and searches (via *thinkering*) for practical, real-world solutions that help us live and grow together in our increasingly complex and recursive world.

What is thinkering? Combine the words *thinking* and *tinkering*. It's an approach to searching and acting that combines all the unique feelings, ideas, beliefs, and reflections that flow through your mind each day with awareness of all the feedback and insights perceived from daily experiences. It is the active pursuit of optimal thought.

how the legendary anchorman Walter Cronkite used to end his broadcasts with, "And that's the way it is." We don't think anyone can say with certainty that any newscast tells you "the way it is" anymore. Those days of "Just the facts, ma'am" (does that also date us?) are long gone. Newscasters are too busy speculating on what might happen or might be true, or just blatantly expressing their opinions, to stick to boring old facts. Inflammatory opinions get better ratings.

Reading is both harder and better for the brain than watching anything on television. If you haven't read a book in a while, you may notice it's a challenge to stay focused at first, but like anything else, the more you read, the easier it becomes and the better your brain gets at paying attention, analyzing, understanding, and remembering. We also watch documentaries—our only TV time—because if we are going to watch television, we want to learn something. But again, discernment is key here. Who funded the documentary? What is the agenda? What are the motives? Who profits from convincing you? We always ask.

The Bigs have figured out how to manipulate our minds and opinions, but vigilance can be your protector. When your mind is strong and independent, you can listen to someone who doesn't agree with you and not get triggered. You can hear someone saying what you hope is true and question it anyway.

> ## PRIMAL WISDOM
>
> There is a huge amount of freedom that comes
> to you when you take nothing personally.
> —DON MIGUEL RUIZ

Respond rather than react. Ask questions: "Why do you think that?" "Where did you hear that?" "How do you know that?" Our favorite question is: "Who told you that story?" because that implies that (1) that information is just a story and (2) that person may be willfully or unintentionally accepting the truth of the story. Or not! If you feel yourself getting angry or upset, ask yourself: "Are they pushing my buttons?" and "Why do I have those buttons?"

Always remember that to react is to be controlled by what someone else is saying. To respond is to maintain control. No matter what you think you know, if you are always willing to listen to an opposing view and consider it critically and with intelligence rather than reacting to it emotionally, then you will have achieved a discerning mind. You will know that the only thing you *can* control is your own response. As Epictetus once wrote, "Any personal capable of angering you becomes your master."

Is It True?

Certainty lies in complete and utter *uncertainty*. Always. Life is complex and full of gray areas. It's easier to side with an extreme because extremes make things simple. It's black or white, hot or cold, light or dark, good or evil. Isn't that convenient? Isn't that easy?

But it's in the middle, in that space between the polarities, where truth lies. The juice between the extremes. "Either/or" is an illusion. We all have our light side and our dark side and every shade in between, and if we don't acknowledge it all, we are living only as a partial person, within an us versus them, person-against-person construct of our culture's making. It's the illusion that you are different and separate from other people.

TAH WHITTY SAYS . . .

Tah Whitty is one of our dearest friends. He hosts the *Mentor in the Mirror* podcast and teaches biointegration along with his wife, Kole.

> Between the extremes of black and white, love and hate, for and against, heaven and hell, is the milky, subtle, and luscious land of the "no-larity." In the "no-larity," there is no attachment, only consideration and exploration. In the absence of attachment, a curious thing happens: Suffering vanishes and ease prevails. In that ease, all things are possible. All points-of-view are just that: simply points-of-view. Nothing to fear, nothing to dread. Nothing to be anxious about. Someone in this space is impossible to control. It's like trying to grasp mercury. Any form of control or oppression is met with a kind of (for the oppressor) maddening mental, spiritual, and emotional Ju-Jitsu.

When you can see that there is a common element within all people, you can finally get to a point where you understand that we're all connected. We're all one, and we're all an expression of each other. What each of us does belongs to all of us, and when you hold all of it and accept and acknowledge all of it, you can see yourself in the face of everyone else on Earth.

That is when you can hold compassion, love, and acceptance for someone and let go of judgment, even if they are "the other." This is the remedy for the division the Bigs try to inflict upon us. This is the medicine for the individual mind as well as the unified collective consciousness.

DAVID NURSE SAYS . . .

Our friend David Nurse, international motivational speaker, author of *Pivot & Go!,* and host of the *Pivot & Go!* podcast, shares these inspirational words about how to think about and talk to yourself about yourself.

> Our biggest obstacle in life is our self. We all wake up with self-doubt, the feeling that we "aren't enough." However, we all have a superhero power inside of us: *choice!* We get the choice to stand in front of the mirror every morning when we wake up and see the foggy mirror of self-doubt, or we can make the choice to wipe away the fog and live in *true* self-awareness of who we were made to be, not who the world is telling us we need to be.

Grappling with Your Own Demons

It's easy for us to say that we should all see the commonality within us and respond rather than react, but in the throes of emotion, we all know this is easier said than done. Whenever we feel like this, we remember a well-known Buddhist parable, which we'll paraphrase here:

> The night before his enlightenment, Siddhartha Gautama struggled with Mara, the demon of doubt, fear, and desire. They argued and wrestled for many hours until finally, both exhausted, Mara went away, and Siddhartha finally attained enlightenment.
>
> After his enlightenment, the Buddha continued to encounter Mara. He often visited, bringing his doubts and fears and temptations. Buddha's loyal assistant, Ananda, was always on the lookout, eager to protect his master from this dark and distracting visitor, but every time he ran to the Buddha to announce, "Mara is coming!" the Buddha just

smiled serenely and said, "I see you Mara. Pull up a cushion and join me for a cup of tea." Mara the demon would sit down and do his worst, but the Buddha would simply listen and watch. Eventually, unable to get a satisfying reaction, Mara would get up and leave. He would never stay for very long.

To acknowledge your doubts, your fears, your knee-jerk reactions, your anger, your desire, is to nullify them. The only way to control your negative reactions is to accept them and choose not to indulge them. You can say, "I see you, fear." "I see you, doubt." "I see you, anger." "I see you, despair." "I see you, feelings of hate for that person I think is wrong." Invite that demon to pull up a cushion and know that it won't take long for it to give up and go away.

What this does is build inner discipline. If you were raised in the Christian tradition, you may remember Jesus's words: "Blessed are the meek, for they shall inherit the earth." This is often interpreted as weak, but meek doesn't mean weak. Translated from the Aramaic, *meek* is more akin to well-trained, or self-controlled. To be meek is to remain unswayed by the fears, doubts, and temptations of the world—to stay steadfast and self-possessed in the face of all that tries to engage you and steal your attention. When you are disciplined, you are in control of your own mind. You don't let anyone steal it.

To tap yet another cultural reference, we once read about the Samurai code: If a Samurai had hate in his heart, he would not kill. He would sooner allow himself to be killed. He would allow himself to kill only when he held love for his enemy in his heart. This may seem paradoxical, but consider whether someone can have the deepest compassion for one's aggressor while still defending life, family, and beliefs. That was the highest of the high ideals—the Samurai gold standard. It is the ultimate in self-possession, the ultimate seeing the self in the other, and it comes only from practice.

It's like anything else. How do you get to the point where you can deadlift five hundred pounds? A few pounds at a time. You start small and you work your way up, with your ideal in your mind.

> ## PRIMAL WISDOM
>
> Hard times create strong men. Strong men create good times.
> Good times create weak men. And weak men create hard times.
> —G. MICHAEL HOPF

None of us are discerning all of the time, but to us, it is the ultimate goal. We need to be discerning to survive. If we want to survive and evolve into the future, we're going to have to reclaim that skill, and there is no time like the present. Don't let them divide and conquer us. Let us rise above that and find our common humanity. When we can do that, no one will be able to take us down.

> ## PRIMAL UPRISING LITMUS TEST
>
> › Should you believe it?
> › Why do you believe it?
> › Who told you that story?
> › What is their motivation? Is there a profit motive? Who profits if you believe what they say?
> › Are they looking to empower you, or keep you captive?
> › Are they telling you to waive your right to information? ("Don't worry about it, we'll take care of everything.")

8

BECOMING MENTALLY RESILIENT

> You have owners. They own you . . . They don't want well-informed, well-educated people capable of critical thinking. They're not interested in that. That doesn't help them. That's against their interests.
>
> —George Carlin

In this world, in this time, it isn't easy to be mentally well and whole. The reason that the first pillar is the physical pillar is that all other pillars of health depend on it, but perhaps none more so than the mental pillar. Your ability to think clearly and with intelligence and discernment is directly linked to your physical health, and poor physical health is a primary cause of poor mental health.

You can see this playing out in actual zoos. Zoo animals often suffer from what appear to be mental illnesses like depression, anxiety, and obsessive-compulsive disorders, for all the reasons we've already talked about. The mismatch between our bodies and brains and our environments have resulted in a similar situation for us. Think about the necessary mental state for hunter-gatherers. They had to be hyperaware, taking in every bit of information from their environment. They lived in the moment, immersed in nature, not constantly distracted. They had to be able to concentrate and make decisions, have discernment and use logic, and communicate with each other clearly and truthfully. They were all in this survival thing together, and they all knew it.

Today, our environments are a far cry from those of our origins. We don't have to pay attention to the world around us to survive, and we have paid a price. We are bombarded with information, much of it irrelevant but taking up space in our brains, and we are rarely able to take a break from it.

When we were being trained recently in the NLP (neuro-linguistic programming) Communication Model, we learned that we are all exposed to 11 million bits of information each second, but we can take in only 126 bits of that 11 million. That's what gets through to us, and we filter it based on our own values, judgments, and behaviors. The rest we delete, distort, or generalize. We create our own internal representation of what we take in, which is why we all have such different versions of reality. Understanding this gives us empathy and compassion for others—we all have the choice to recognize that each person perceives reality a bit differently, and that's normal.

PRIMAL WISDOM

Just as a gardener cultivates his plot, keeping it free
from weeds, and growing the flowers and fruits which he
requires, so may a man tend the garden of his mind.
—JAMES ALLEN

The Brain Fog Diet

Because mental health starts with physical health, it makes sense to lay a foundation for mental health with food. First, what is harmful? When it comes to brain health, there are two primary food ingredients that are the most likely to have a damaging effect on your brain: sugar (especially fructose) and gluten (especially in wheat).[15] Sugar and gluten are ubiquitous, addictive, damaging, and totally legal, and have caused tremendous amounts of pain, suffering, and poor health. Refined sugar is as addictive as cocaine (there is a reason why they call it "the white death").[16] It's also implicated in the development of insulin resistance, which can lead to dementia. Some experts now call Alzheimer's disease "type 3 diabetes." As for wheat, one study demonstrated that wheat bread increases gut permeability, which can lead to brain-damaging autoimmune reactions, and contains opioid-like qualities that can cause "mental derangement."[17] The thousands of foods that contain both sugar and gluten (doughnuts, cookies, muffins, cakes, the aforementioned bread, and so on) are an irresistible dopamine hit to the brain.

We now have young children with measurably clogged arteries, diabetes, and brain plaque. We *know it hurts our brains and harms our children,* and yet we keep right on eating it. We think we "can't stop" drinking soda, eating candy, or binging on cookies, but that's just a story that comes with a side of guilt and self-loathing.

The only way to free yourself is to stop. Just stop, cold turkey. Step away from the bread, the pasta, the plate of cookies, the breakroom muffins, the office candy jar. Quitting sugar and gluten is damn excruciating at first, but when you finally step out of your fog and look back, you'll wonder why you ever ate them. You won't believe the clarity of thought you can achieve. We've done it, and so have many of our friends. It *is* possible to go "against the grain."

Some tools to help: Your conscious mind is the goal setter and the unconscious mind is the goal getter, so be careful what you say about yourself ("I can't quit sugar," "I love bread too much," "I have no willpower"). What we tell the unconscious mind shapes belief. You can use this to your advantage. Michelle recently learned an NLP technique to help her stop eating ice cream at night. Her trainer asked her where she visualized ice cream. She said she imagined it right in front of her. Then the trainer asked where she visualized the food she loathes most: lima beans. She said she saw them way over to her left. The trainer asked her to visualize taking the ice cream and moving it behind the lima beans, then putting them in a bag and shaking it all up together. Now, whenever Michelle thinks of ice cream, all she can see is a disgusting mess of ice cream–covered lima beans. That siren song of ice cream has suddenly become manageable. Change the mindset, change your words, and be free.

THE GUT-BRAIN CONNECTION

The community of microbes—mostly bacteria but also fungi and viruses—that live in the digestive tract have a direct line to the brain through hormone and neuronal signaling along the vagus nerve, from the brain to the gut and back, called the gut-brain axis. This connection is responsible for nervous stomachs, "butterflies," and the reason why people with digestive disorders like irritable bowel syndrome (IBS) can experience related neurological issues like anxiety. What you eat influences which microbes thrive or don't.

We know that fiber promotes the growth of beneficial bacteria and sugar promotes the growth of pathogenic fungi. Since beneficial microbes in your gut help manufacture most of your body's serotonin (the hormone that contributes to a good mood and feelings of happiness), taking care of your microbiome is a critical component of mental health.

To keep that "gut garden" well fertilized, eat as many vegetables as you can every day, including fermented veggies that are already growing their own beneficial bacteria. Your good microbes also like the polyphenols in fresh berries.

Building a Better Brain

Many other lifestyle factors besides food influence mental health, but you can boil them all down to providing the human brain with a more natural human environment. Here are the most important environmental and lifestyle shifts you can make to positively impact mental health.

Sleep better

Research has shown that seven hours per night is the minimum amount of sleep necessary to support cognitive function.[18] The amount of time spent in different stages of sleep is also important. Compromised REM sleep (the rapid eye movement stage of sleep during which dreaming typically occurs) is associated with both depression and anxiety as well as lower cognitive function, and a lack of sufficient deep sleep is associated with dementia. Scientists only recently discovered that the brain and central nervous system have their own lymphatic system for waste removal, called the glymphatic system, and that it works most efficiently to restore brain health during deep sleep by flushing out neural waste that could otherwise accumulate and lead to the plaques and tangles associated with dementia.[19]

Improving your sleep hygiene will improve your sleep quality and, by extension, your mental health. Wind down an hour or two before bed by doing relaxing things. Keep televisions and other screens out of your bedroom. Don't eat or exercise too close to bedtime. Try to go to sleep and wake up at around the same time every day, including on weekends. Synch your wake-up time with sunrise, as much as possible, and expose yourself to more natural lighting. If you need help relaxing, a melatonin and/or high-quality magnesium supplement could help.

There are many sleep trackers out there to help you understand your sleep length and quality. One of our favorites is the Oura Ring, which tracks your time in light sleep, REM sleep, and deep sleep, as well as your temperature and respiration rate during the night. (It has a very low level of electromagnetic field transmission compared to some sleep trackers, so we feel it's safe to wear while sleeping, and we are both people who turn our phones on airplane mode at night.) It also tells you your activity level during the day, and gives you a sleep score and readiness score, to help you determine whether you should go hard when you slept well, or take it easy after a night of low-quality sleep.

Naturalize your lighting

Before the invention of electric lights, humans encountered full-spectrum light during the day when the sun was up, but only light on the red end of the spectrum after dark, from firelight. Disrupting this biological expectation disrupts the sleep-wake cycle (circadian rhythm), compromising sleep length and quality. Computers, televisions, and other screens (such as on smartphones) emit blue light, which can suppress the release of melatonin, the hormone that triggers sleepiness.

Many people aren't willing to put away their phones or turn off their televisions at sundown, but most smartphones now have a night mode that blocks the blue light for you. You can also hack your way to a more natural light experience with blue light–blocking glasses. Our friend Dave Asprey makes a nice line of these glasses called TrueDark (there are other good brands, too). He says that too much blue light at night can cause inflammation that's linked to a host of chronic diseases, including cancer, diabetes, and vision loss. By putting on blue light–blocking glasses as soon as the sun sets, you help your brain release melatonin to ease you more naturally into sleep.

In the morning, you can also make yourself feel more awake if you step outside into the sunlight for a few minutes, to trigger cortisol, which helps you wake up and get ready for the day. Imagine you are stepping out of your cave and considering your plan for gathering your breakfast. (While you're at it, you can actually plan a more natural breakfast. Berries and nuts? A couple of eggs and some greens?)

Move more

Brains need oxygen, circulation, and stimulation, so it makes sense that moving improves brain function. This is supported by research. There are hundreds (thousands?) of studies on the effects of exercise on mental health, and there is no doubt that regular exercise improves mental health. A famous study showed cardiovascular exercise (like running) to be just as effective a treatment for depression as antidepressant medication.[20] Another study showed that adding more physical activity back into elementary schools dramatically improved learning.[21] Keith's elementary school teachers used to send Keith outside to run around for a few minutes, to help him stop fidgeting and pay attention. It always worked!

Exercise is most effective at alleviating mental health issues at about forty-five minutes a day, with a frequency of three to five times per week.[22] We've already talked in detail about exercise, so we won't go through physical pillar basics again—we hope you are already working on that. Just consider this another significant benefit of exercise, especially outdoors.

Go outside

We evolved outdoors, which is probably a big part of why most people feel better when they go outside, especially in areas with lots of trees and/or water. Going outside on a sunny day also feels good because sun helps the body manufacture vitamin D.[23] Most people in the US are deficient in vitamin D, and research shows that low vitamin D is linked to depression and other mental disorders, as well as many other chronic health conditions.[24] Getting outside delivers vitamin D the natural way, but most of us still can't get enough so we recommend taking a vitamin D3 supplement (along with vitamin K2, which helps vitamin D work better).

Focus

Brains can learn to be distracted and can learn to focus. To teach yours to focus, carve out periods of time during the day when you do not allow yourself to get distracted by a pinging phone, emails or texts, social media, or wandering to the refrigerator to find something to eat. The internet is probably the greatest time suck ever known to humankind. It's junk food for the mind. The dopamine-hits people get with every "like" and "follow" makes distraction feel addictive. The more you make yourself focus, the easier it gets. (We refer you to our discussion of the Pomodoro Technique on page 91.)

Manage stress

Finances, relationships, family, work, the state of the world—it's all stressful, but learning how to manage and grow from stress is how we survived as a species. *We know how to do this,* but what we tend to forget is that the benefits of stress happen during recovery from that stress.

Imagine a gazelle on the savanna. Gazelles are alert but calm most of the time, grazing in groups. They don't stand around fretting that they are probably going to get eaten. However, when a lion pops out of the brush and starts the chase, the gazelle kicks into high gear and runs for its life. As soon as the threat is gone (the lion got the other guy), the gazelles go back to grazing.

This is an example of how the nervous system works. When gazelles (or humans) are calm and relaxed, going about their business, the parasympathetic nervous system ("rest and digest" mode) is in charge. When something stressful happens, the brain switches over to the sympathetic nervous system, sending signals to the body to pump out stress hormones like cortisol and adrenaline, for greater speed, strength, and quick reactions. Once the threat is past, the parasympathetic mode should take over again.

If you think of yourself like the gazelle, and your stress (the job you don't like, your money situation, your family issues, your relationship problems, or whatever it is) as the lion, you can see how unnatural it would be to run from the lion 24-7, even when there is no lion in sight. Sustained levels of those stress hormones increase inflammation and can lead to chronic disease. You should be in grazing mode *most of the time.* Even if you meditate for twenty minutes at the end of the day, those few minutes of meditation can't make up for twelve hours of high stress. It should be the other way around.

Let's say you have to get up in front of people and talk. You could worry about it all day, or you could let your body kick into sympathetic nervous system mode only while you are up there in front of the audience, so you can use those sharpened senses for better performance. Be the gazelle.

Easier said than done, of course. Learning not to worry all day is a skill, and mental resilience helps you use your brain the way you want to use it. Resilient minds can concentrate, relax, make decisions, and be creative whenever they want to be.

There is a mental game for this mental problem: The secret to a life in parasympathetic mode is to separate out what you can't control (most things) and let them go, while focusing your energy on what you can control (your own actions and reactions). This is daily work and a long game, but it will literally change your mind.

To support that effort, you can also use stress "dosing" to strengthen your mental capacity. Here are some ways to train by purposefully exposing your mind to effort, then balancing it with recovery. When it counts, these exercises will help you be the one in control, not the lion.

PRIMAL WISDOM

Humans are the only species that can have a thought and change the entire chemical makeup of their bodies.
—CHRISTOPHER SHADE

Challenges

Try to do at least one of these every day:

- **Play hard.** Play brain games to tax different parts of your brain, like memory, speed, attention, and flexibility, or do word or number puzzles.
- **Play smart.** Play strategy games like chess or poker (check out the great book *Thinking in Bets* by Annie Duke).
- **Think and move.** Combine strategy with movement, as in rock climbing. Keith and Michelle like to hike with their dogs in a nearby dry creek bed strewn with large rocks. Every step must be calculated.
- **Argue.** Argue a set of statistics, without altering any numbers or results, from opposite points of view.
- **Point and counterpoint.** The next time you read an essay or opinion piece, find and read a counterpoint, to get both sides.

- **Remember.** The next time you are trying to remember something, don't look it up on your phone. Give yourself five minutes to remember it yourself.

- **Memorize.** Commit things to memory: your favorite poem, people's phone numbers, song lyrics, or anything else. If all technology disappeared tomorrow, what would you want to be able to remember?

- **Write it out.** Write in a journal every day. Keep track of what you do, what you are thinking about, or what you are grateful for.

- **Learn something new.** Start learning a new language with online or audiobook lessons, or refresh that language you studied in high school. Pick up a musical instrument like the guitar, piano, ukulele, recorder, or harmonica.

- **Use a map** to get somewhere instead of your GPS. Or take it to the next level by learning orienteering, a cool sport that requires navigating over difficult, unfamiliar terrain as fast as possible, using only a map and a compass.

- **Learn a new vocabulary word** every day.

- **Buy a used textbook** on a subject that interests you and read it. Do the study exercises.

- **Research** and learn all about something that interests you.

ABEL JAMES SAYS . . .

Our friend Abel James is the host of the *Fat-Burning Man* podcast and the author of *The Wild Diet* and *Designer Babies Still Get Scabies*. We agree with his take on mental wellness:

> When our mental health and basic needs of survival are threatened, it's time to get focused. As the threat level escalates to red, it's tempting to think that "checking the news and social media is more important than meditating," but this is exactly when we need to prioritize mental balance more than ever.

- **Do something creative** every day. Exercising your creativity has great mental expansion powers. Draw, write, dance, paint, make collages or vision boards, make up stories, take photographs, envision and plan a new business, house, or a new you.
- **Live on the edge.** If you want to go super edgy, experiment with microdosing. See pages 121–122.

Recoveries

To balance the challenge, you need recovery. Try to do at least one of these every day:

- **Sleep it off.** Go to bed an hour earlier.
- **Meditate on it.** Meditation is an ancient and proven technique for increasing brain power, memory, cognition, and clarity of thought. There is a huge body of research supporting its physical and mental benefits.[25] There are many meditation techniques and they all work. Here are some techniques to try:
  - › Pay attention to the sound and feel of your breath moving in and out.
  - › Focus mindfully on your surroundings.
  - › Repeat a calming word (known as a mantra) out loud or in your head.
  - › Visualize a peaceful scene or imagine yourself in a place that makes you happy.
  - › Just sit and relax your mind, letting thoughts come and go but not engaging with them.

  Meditate for fifteen minutes in the morning and fifteen minutes at night. There are many helpful apps to get you started; Sam Harris's meditation app Waking Up is a great resource for this. We also like the Muse headband device, which gamifies meditation and teaches you how to get your brain waves to do what you want.

- **Stretch through it.** Do thirty minutes of yoga.
- **Hypnotize yourself.** We use NLP self-hypnotic techniques for both performance and recovery.
- **Put a positive spin on it.** Michelle uses positive affirmations every day. She says them to herself in the present tense "as if now," beginning with "I receive and believe and I'm so grateful for . . ." She has about fifty affirmations she says daily in the morning and evening.
- **Work it out.** Do any exercise. This is Keith's go-to for stress management. His favorite way to handle stress is to exhaust the lower body. You can do this any way you choose, from running to squats.
- **Shake it off.** Shaking is a way to process trauma and can also ease anxiety and restore focus. Keith likes to use a technique developed by Dr. David Berceli, which we'll tell you how to do in the resources section at PrimalUprising.com/BookResources.
- **Enjoy yourself.** Read a book you love or listen to your favorite music.
- **Zone out.** Do absolutely nothing for five minutes. Just sit there. (Hard at first, until it becomes amazing.)
- **Query it.** Close your eyes, take a few deep breaths, then ask yourself the question that has been bothering you. Clear your mind and wait. Often, the answer is right at the subconscious level and will come to the surface.
- **Tap your tribe.** There is nothing more natural and stress-relieving than talking to the people who understand you best, whether that's family or friends. Just being with other people can help, even if you never mention your stress.
- **Breathe.** Try a breathwork technique—breathing exercises can almost immediately reverse the stress response. Some options:
  › Breathe slowly and deeply for five minutes.
  › Try the 4-7-8 breathing technique (popularized by Dr. Andrew Weil): Place the tip of your tongue just behind your front teeth. Exhale fully, then inhale through your nose for four seconds,

hold your breath for seven seconds, and exhale forcefully through your mouth for eight seconds. Do this four times.

> Practice the yoga technique with pranayama. A yoga teacher can guide you.

BEN GREENFIELD SAYS ...

Our friend Ben Greenfield, author of *Boundless*, is always pushing the envelope to see what his body and brain can do. He is a big advocate of breathwork. Here's what he says about its benefits:

It turns out breathwork is about more than conscious activation of your immune system. The expansive list of benefits (just to name a few) include nitric oxide production, CO_2 retention, mental clarity, aerobic capacity, decreased salivary and plasma cortisol, and faster sleep onset.

Cognitive Enhancement

Once you've got your mental health and stress management going in the right direction, you can go up from a healthy baseline to make yourself smarter, sharper, and quicker. In the movie *Limitless,* the actor Bradley Cooper's character discovers a drug that instantly dials up his intelligence, alertness, motivation, and charisma. It turns him into a genius. Who wouldn't be drawn to such a thing? There's been a lot of cutting-edge research and experimentation into this area. We have discovered that some substances really do increase cognitive function. Some are legal and ubiquitous, like caffeine. Keith is a big fan, and drinks it all day long, while Michelle has one perfect cup of coffee in the morning.

Some substances are demonized but used anyway, like nicotine. While we all agree that smoking isn't good for anyone, microdosing with patches, gum, nicotine lozenges, or sublingual spray can sharpen cognition. (Vaping is better than smoking, but it's not a clean nicotine delivery system, and we don't yet fully understand the risks involved.) We both like the mental sharpness we get from the occasional hit of nicotine.

Some other smart drugs are available by prescription only, like Modafinil (allegedly the drug on which *Limitless* was based). When Keith was in the military, he took Modafinil like candy to stay awake and alert for twenty-four, thirty-six, or forty-eight hours, whenever that was required. Keith will tell you that it works as advertised, but the crash afterward is horrible, and he hopes he never has to experience it again. Some people use ADHD drugs like Adderall off-label to focus on an important task. It's notoriously used by students to help them study, but ADHD drugs can be habit-forming.

These substances all have their place, for those who want to experiment with them (although we don't advise doing anything illegal). Many people microdose these substances, meaning they take very small doses to get a tiny boost without impairment or addiction.

A more controversial practice is microdosing LSD or psilocybin. We do this for cognitive enhancement and a more attuned awareness. There is a sweet spot between feeling nothing and achieving expanded awareness without actually perceiving a hallucinogenic effect.

TAKE IT TO THE NEXT LEVEL WITH PLANT AND ANIMAL MEDICINES

Naturally derived medicines from cannabis to ayahuasca to Bufo toad venom intimidate many people, but under the guidance of an experienced and reputable shaman or guide, these substances can blow open parts of consciousness that would otherwise be difficult to access (although some can get the same effect from high-level meditation). These are powerful therapies for resolving trauma and increasing self-awareness. We'll explore them more in chapter 12.

Once you've consciously engaged your mental health, you can move on to the next level: emotional wellness.

PRIMAL UPRISING LITMUS TEST

> What are the ways I challenge my mind? Could I do this more?
> What are the ways I allow my mind to recover? Could I do this more?
> Do I meditate? Do I do it consistently?
> Do I manage my stress enough that it doesn't affect my health? (Am I sure?)
> Would I ever try cognitive enhancers? What would my reasons be?

PART IV
THE
EMOTIONAL
PILLAR

Your eyes can deceive you. Don't trust them. Stretch out with your feelings!

—Obi-Wan Kenobi (from *Star Wars Episode IV: A New Hope*)

9

FREE TO FEEL

Thought is deeper than all speech,
Feeling deeper than all thought.

—Christopher Pearse Cranch

We are emotional beings, and emotions are part of the human experience. In fact, emotion is what makes human consciousness such an incredibly vast terrain to explore. It's unfortunate that our culture generally puts a negative connotation on "being emotional." It's seen as either a weakness (especially in men—"Big boys don't cry") or a sign of unreliability (especially in women—"Hysterical woman!"). It's neither, of course. We all express emotions differently, and all ways are valid. Emotions become a problem only when we refuse to acknowledge them, or when we let them carry us away into extreme behavior that hurts us or others.

To be emotionally intelligent is to be the one in charge of your emotions, rather than having your emotions be in charge of you, respond rather than react, understand and actually accept how you feel, fully feel something without letting the feelings make you do things you wouldn't do when in a more logical frame of mind, and understand and be sensitive to the emotions of others. What's not emotionally intelligent is to lose your temper, say or do things in the heat of the moment, quit something out of frustration, or deny and repress how you feel.

In the next chapter, we'll get into some specific strategies for how to work on emotional intelligence, but in this chapter, we want to talk about emotions in terms of gender. This is something we've both struggled with and had some pretty big realizations about. Is it politically correct? Probably not, but if you know us, you know we're going to go there anyway.

Gendered Feelings

Gender is a controversial subject. Is it biological or cultural? Actually, it's both. Women and men process and experience emotions differently in some ways (although obviously not all ways), and it's largely because of hormones. Research bears out that men, with more testosterone, are more likely to contend with aggression, and women, with more estrogen and life stages that include hormonal fluctuation, are more likely to contend with mood swings.[26]

Culturally, gender roles used to be prescribed for purposes of survival. Men (generally) have an aggressive instinct that made them good at hunting. Women (generally) have a maternal instinct that made them good at raising the children and nurturing the tribe. Yet, research on gender roles in the Paleolithic era indicate that in many cases, hunter-gatherers were more egalitarian than previously believed. Men and women had different jobs but were considered equally valuable for the survival of the tribe.[27] Some surmise that this changed with the dawn of agriculture, when women became property.[28] Just one more reason to embrace a paleo lifestyle—equal rights! Let's use that as a jumping-off point.

Our culture constantly and obsessively assigns qualities to men versus women. It's like we can't help it. It starts young, with pink and blue baby clothes and accessories. We have a pink aisle and a blue aisle in the toy store. We use different compliments (pretty versus handsome) and different insults (bitch versus asshole—try analyzing that one!). We can guarantee that if someone androgynous-looking walks into a room, the first thing on most people's minds will be to wonder: *Is that a man or a woman?* Rude, yes, but it's a reality, right or wrong. We are gender-obsessed.

To some extent, we think this is founded on the real difference in feminine and masculine energy. Ancient cultures recognized this dichotomy—male and female, light and dark, sun and moon, yin and yang—and knew that both ends were necessary for balance. The best version of a man doesn't mean the absence of feminine energy, but a balance in which feminine energy bolsters male energy. The best version of a woman doesn't mean the absence of masculine energy, but a balance in which masculine energy bolsters feminine energy. In fact, a "best masculine" cannot exist in the absence of a "best feminine" to match it, or (as they say these days) hold space for it. And vice versa.

But like so many other things, we have taken our gender obsession too far. We confuse gender shadow sides with what should be healthy integrated expressions of spiritual energy (we'll talk more about this in the Spirituality Pillar). Toxic masculinity encompasses feelings and actions like bullying, offensive rather than defensive violence, cat-calling, subjugation of women, sexual assault or harassment, and the idea that this is just "boys being boys," rather than the unintegrated shadow side of the male energy. This has become confused with regular masculinity. We all have our shadow sides, men and women both. Somehow though, we have managed to either tolerate toxicity masculinity—"a man's right to be a man"—or demonize it as something that shouldn't exist at all, or that should be repressed, rather than something that should be observed, recognized, and then integrated.

For women, being emotional has become confused with femininity, but that isn't right either. Extreme irrational emotion is a shadow side of all humans, not just women, but it's expressed differently in both genders. When men submit to their extreme emotions, the result is more likely (but not always) physical violence. When women submit to their extreme emotions, the result may be physical violence, but it is more likely (or more stereotypically) related to mood swings, or quickly shifting emotions. It's acceptable for women to be more emotional from birth—or it might be more correct to say that men are encouraged *not* to be emotional from birth, whereas women aren't usually saddled with the burden of suppressing emotion. Women are, however, often expected to take responsibility for other people's emotions, often ahead of their own.

The first thing to recognize is that there is no black-and-white to any of this. There are exceptions, and degrees, and a spectrum. However, understanding how gender might be influencing your emotional struggles can be useful. (And yes, of course this applies to anyone of any gender identification; no matter how you identify, you have—or take—hormones.)

Let's dig in to how these gender expressions and emotions can affect people in their everyday lives.

"There's No Crying in Baseball!"

Michelle has contended with the issue of gender and emotion ever since she became the CEO of Paleo f(x). In this leadership role, she thought she had to act like a man to be taken seriously. Who would listen to an emotional woman? That famous line from the movie *A League of Their Own* comes to mind, when baseball manager Jimmy Dugan (played by Tom Hanks) doesn't know how to handle a team of women, and when one of the women cries after he yells at her, he doesn't understand her emotional response. He says, "There's no crying in baseball. *There's no crying in baseball!*" (Which makes her cry harder.)

Michelle believed there was no crying in business, and that she had to steel herself to be a good CEO. She didn't have a role model for a woman CEO, and she didn't know what leadership looked like from a strong feminine perspective, but she had her own preconceptions of how male CEOs would act. That was her blueprint, but it made interacting with others feel unnatural. Instead of getting respected for behaving aggressively, Michelle got called a bitch, so she did everything herself. She didn't trust others to do things the right way. Paleo f(x) is a huge event with thousands of moving parts, and Michelle was managing every speaker, contractor, exhibitor, and venue. When the event and the company grew beyond what one person could manage, Michelle had to admit she needed help. Together we sat down and made a plan to delegate the work to a team, but this was a difficult transition for Michelle. She didn't trust the team, and she was overly critical.

This made people not want to work for her. Michelle can honestly say that she ran off a lot of employees because she didn't let people own their own jobs. She thought she was being strong ("masculine"), but she was driving them all crazy.

Whenever the team came to her with a problem and an idea to make things better, she took it personally. She was offended by the implied criticism.

To figure this out, Michelle had to find her feminine energy and she found it in her "mama bear" side. She realized Paleo f(x) was like a child to her, especially since it was created as a legacy in honor of her daughter Brittani. She saw that she was going to have to take her ego out of it and recognize that the team really did want to make the event the best it could be. She had to trust them.

Michelle gathered her team and told them: "Please understand that when you come to me with an idea, come to me with the idea. Leave out the part about everything we did wrong previously because to me, that's like you're telling me my baby is ugly. It makes me feel like a horrible mother to this company. Tell me how you are making the baby more successful."

Michelle found a photo of a baby graphically merged with a dog to create an admittedly pretty disturbing picture, and whenever the team began to lapse into any kind of talk about how something with Paleo f(x) wasn't working, she held up the picture and they knew to back off and change course—no insulting the baby! This helped the team communicate better with Michelle, and it changed the whole company. When she began to allow them to do what they loved and were good at, she ended up with something much better than she could ever have done by herself.

Michelle realizes now that she never actually wanted control. She wanted influence. Control breeds resentment. Influence builds loyalty. She began to navigate her position of authority as herself, not as some idea of how CEOs are supposed to act, and life got better for everyone. It's stressful to try to be someone you're not. Now, it doesn't matter to her how they get to the end result as long as they create her vision of the event or better.

To be a good leader is to balance the masculine and feminine while operating from that authentic place of *you*, beyond stereotypes. That place will likely be influenced by gender, but first and foremost it will be influenced by your personality and your emotional life. Today, although Michelle didn't have good female leadership role models, she has become one for others. And if she needs to cry, she'll cry.

LISA WHITTY BRADLEY, MD, FACS, SAYS . . .

Our friend Lisa Whitty Bradley, CEO and founder of Chicks with MDs, LLC, and a bestselling author under the pseudonym Stella Jones, says this about confidence:

> The world uses what it perceives as your weakness to attempt to deter and deflate you. Being an African American woman has always been my ace in the hole. When I speak with pre-med students and doctors, I often tell them what I remind myself when faced with adversaries who try to limit me because of their preconceived notions about my sex, race, or "disability": Their opinion of me is not my business! You are the rate-limiting step in your success. Your path is determined by the person you face when you wake up every single morning of your life.

The Warrior in the Garden

Just as many women struggle with how to navigate leadership positions with healthy feminine energy, many men struggle with how to navigate more supportive or traditionally female roles with healthy masculine energy. Imagine the husband of a woman who is a CEO. If they have children, he may choose to stay home with them and be the "house husband." Maybe a man works for a company with a woman as his boss. Maybe a man makes less money than his wife. It may be a cultural bias, but it can feel emasculating nevertheless. (Although we have to acknowledge that while a woman CEO is often called a bitch, a house husband is often celebrated for every little accomplishment. "Look! He changed a diaper! What a great dad!")

Being in a supportive role can be challenging for men if they think they need to act like a woman would act, when that isn't authentic to their nature. Men in support roles need to find that line between being fully in their masculine energy and accessing their feminine energy to be caretakers or support systems. A man won't parent or keep house or be on support staff exactly the way a woman would, just as a woman won't lead the way a man would. Both should embrace their roles in a way that is authentic to them. For a man, emotional intelligence means not feeling emasculated by taking care of children or cleaning the kitchen, but understanding his role in the context of his individual life and relationship.

Not all men would want to do this, just as not all women would want to be CEOs, but we live in a world where anyone can be anything, so we need to adapt our emotional intelligence to that reality. It's not the job that dictates the gender, but the gender that (partially) dictates the way someone does the job.

Keith struggled with this for a long time because he is not comfortable in a CEO type of position. Leadership isn't how Keith operates, or wants to operate. This is complicated for a guy who is devoted to the paleo lifestyle and is always looking to hunter-gatherers for direction, but Keith also recognizes that one of the benefits of modern life is that we don't have to be beholden to those roles if they don't fit with our personalities. We no longer have that ecological pressure for prescribed roles based on survival needs. We can all do what we do best, gender aside. We once might have needed the strong men to drag home the buffalo, but anyone can go to the grocery store and buy a package of steak.

It took a lot of emotional work, but Keith finally discovered that if Paleo f(x) were a ship at sea, he wanted to be—and felt most at home and most capable—holding the sextant, interpreting the map, scanning the seas and the weather, and helping plot the course. How the ship got there—all the doings of "business"—bored him. But locating the destination! *That* was exciting! Now he feels like he plays an important role that is also authentic to his personality and energy.

BARBARA DITLOW SAYS . . .

Human Design is a system that helps people understand themselves better. It has transformed our work and personal lives. Knowing what is innate and unchangeable for you can help you claim and embrace your qualities rather than fighting against them or trying to change what is essential to your nature. One hour with a good coach can set you on the path to emotional intelligence and inner harmony. Barbara Ditlow is our Human Design analyst, teacher, and coach. She has helped us understand ourselves and each other in ways we don't think we otherwise could have. Here are her thoughts on Human Design:

> Human Design is nothing short of miraculous. As a synthesis of esoteric and exoteric knowledge, its practical decision-making process reveals an entirely different dimension from which decisions can be made. For me as well as those with whom I share this knowledge, it provides a unique individualized blueprint for awakening.

Find links to learn more about human Human Design at the Resources webpage at PrimalUprising.com/BookResources.

We'll leave you with an image that we think best represents emotional intelligence: If you were to spin a top on a table, it may look like it is spinning in perfect balance, but if you were to watch the top under magnification, you'd see that it's wobbling constantly to stay upright. It's making micro-adjustments all the time, until it runs out of energy and falls over. To stay in balance with your emotions, with your femininity and masculinity, and to be able to feel and process your emotions without spinning right over the edge of the table requires constant micro-adjustments. You can live in awareness of how you feel rather than in denial. You can respond rather than react. You can know yourself and be in tune with others. You can behave like a human being, in all your emotional complexity, without misbehaving or feeling like you are at the mercy of your emotional ebbs and flows.

Next we'll look at how to build emotional resilience so you can master emotional intelligence.

PRIMAL UPRISING LITMUS TEST

> Are your feminine and masculine sides balanced?
> How could you get comfortable with both?
> Do you acknowledge your shadow side? Are you capable of controlling it?
> What role do you play in your relationships, work life, and personal life?
> Do you feel authentic in those roles?

10

BECOMING EMOTIONALLY RESILIENT

One loses the capacity to grieve as a child grieves, or to rage as a child rages: hotly, despairingly, with tears of passion. One grows up, one becomes civilized, one learns one's manners, and consequently can no longer manage these two functions—sorrow and anger—adequately.

—Anita Brookner

Imagine feeling a strong emotion, like anger, fear, or intense joy, and letting yourself feel it fully but not get carried away by it. It sounds easy, but it's the work of a lifetime. Somehow, we knew how to do it when we were young, and somehow, we forgot.

One of the meditation techniques we appreciate is letting emotions move through the body and mind with full awareness but without reactivity or attachment—to be the watcher of the feelings, rather than engaging with them and letting them distract and manipulate.

You can do this when you aren't meditating, but it takes some practice to let feelings flow through you, completely felt but put into perspective. They are just feelings. They are important, but they do not define you. You can say: "I feel XYZ" versus "I *am* XYZ." In a moment (or a day, or a month, or a year), the feelings will be gone, but you will remain you.

This makes it possible to feel anger without lashing out, feel fear without running away, and feel joy without, for example, getting married after a spectacular first date. This is different than denying emotion, which would be to deny your own humanity. Emotional resilience makes this distinction possible. Without it, you may have trouble feeling the feeling, or you may fear or dread the feeling. Either can result in repressing the feeling or acting irrationally because of it. Emotional resilience also means taking 100 percent responsibility for every emotion you experience, rather than blaming someone else for "causing" your emotions. When you don't own your emotions but blame them on someone or something else, you cede your sovereignty to an "other."

Emotional resilience, like every other kind of resilience, is about adaptability. You can ride the highs and the lows, the agony and the ecstasy, the joy and the sorrow, the waves of human emotion at their most dramatic, without getting tossed about or drawn under, and you can take full responsibility for all of it. In this chapter, we'll talk about some ways to practice this, so you can learn to understand and manage your own emotions.

PRIMAL WISDOM

Offense is taken, not given. No need to disarm the world. Just make yourself bulletproof. Sticks and stones, people. Block. Unfollow. Laugh.
—RICKY GERVAIS (ON TWITTER)

Trigger Warning

Let's talk about getting triggered. (Yeah, we're going to go there!) To be triggered is to experience an intense emotion because of what someone else says. If you are triggered, it's usually because you have had a traumatic personal experience and someone has reminded you of it (often inadvertently), and this takes you back to that traumatic feeling. You can find trigger warnings all over social media these days because whenever someone talks about something that might possibly trigger someone about something, they want to make sure that person has the chance to avoid getting triggered.

The sentiment behind trigger warnings is compassion, and that's a good thing. If you know someone lost a loved one to cancer, it would be insensitive to make a joke about cancer in front of that person. If you know someone was battered or abused, you don't make jokes or tell stories about someone being battered or abused. It's not polite or compassionate to trigger someone. That's just being a good person.

But like everything else in our culture, this whole triggering business has gone way too far. We don't want to be insensitive, but now everybody is so overly afraid to offend anybody about anything that we've practically muzzled ourselves. There is a line somewhere between compassion and walking on eggshells. And, since you can't control what other people do or say anyway, why not take action to protect yourself instead? There will always be rude, inconsiderate people out there, but most of us are doing our best to get along and act like good humans. Instead of policing everybody's words all the time, we think we would all be better served by practicing emotional resilience.

To be triggered is to be emotionally reactive, but it's a knee-jerk reaction and can turn dangerous. Look at what happens with riots and mob mentality—it's the result of one big infectious trigger. It's heightened, highly reactive, explosive emotion in motion. There is no calculated response by a mob. It's all just feelings gone wild.

But on the personal level, apart from the mob, when it's just you and your feelings, this is something you can work on for yourself. We all feel strong feelings. We have all gone through some bad, even traumatic experiences, but the fact is that we can never fully control what other people do. We can only control ourselves, and that means we can control, at least eventually, with practice, how easily we are triggered.

Every time you get triggered, you have an opportunity to practice resilience: To fully feel the feeling and work on learning to separate who you are from what you feel. You can feel it without acting on it or being defined by it. Invite that triggering feeling to sit down and have tea with you, like the Buddha did with Mara. Get to know it, but don't let it carry you away. When it has outstayed its welcome, it will leave. It may also help to remember that what you are feeling is related to something that happened to you, but it was just something that happened to you. It isn't you.

THE HEART'S ENERGY

According to Rollin McCraty, psychophysiologist with the HeartMath Institute, the magnetic energy of the heart is five thousand times stronger than the magnetic energy emanating from the brain. In his article "The Resonant Heart," he writes:[29]

> Basic research at the Institute of HeartMath shows that information pertaining to a person's emotional state is also communicated throughout the body via the heart's electromagnetic field. The rhythmic beating patterns of the heart change significantly as we experience different emotions. Negative emotions, such as anger or frustration, are associated with an erratic, disordered, incoherent pattern in the heart's rhythms. In contrast, positive emotions, such as love or appreciation, are associated with a smooth, ordered, coherent pattern in the heart's rhythmic activity. In turn, these changes in the heart's beating patterns create corresponding changes in the structure of the electromagnetic field radiated by the heart, measurable by a technique called spectral analysis. More specifically, we have demonstrated that sustained positive emotions appear to give rise to a distinct mode of functioning, which we call psychophysiological coherence. During this mode, heart rhythms exhibit a sine wave-like pattern and the heart's electromagnetic field becomes correspondingly more organized.

McCraty also posits that this electromagnetic energy extends up to five feet beyond the human body. This may be what we feel when we feel the energy of another human who is standing next to us. Step back six feet and you lose that connection.

Part of learning how not to get triggered is to stop judging your emotions. Judgment only brings about shame and guilt and the need to hide who you are. When you no longer judge yourself or others for your emotions, they can become just another part of the natural human experience. Emotions aren't good, bad, or indifferent. They just are. See them, feel them, know them, and know that you can choose not to let them control your words or actions. This takes work, but it's worthwhile work because there's no winning in judgment. There's no freedom in shame. There's no responsibility in lashing out, and there is no peace in regret.

When you think that you are your emotions, then it's easier to justify bad behavior. It's like the parent who hits a child and says, "Look what you made me do." When you can separate your emotions from yourself, you can realize you are responsible for what you do. You don't have to give power to the feeling. You have the power.

Another trigger for many people occurs when someone projects something onto them, calling them a name or making assumptions about them. This can create an emotion inside someone because they feel judged, like when Michelle thought that her staff's ideas were personal attacks on our business. But the thing is, the projection isn't yours. It belongs to the person who projected it. When you start to realize that you never have to react to somebody else's projection, and that to do so gives that person power and allows them to control you, then you will see that your emotional reaction is keeping you captive. You're at the mercy of someone else's emotional fluctuations. You're not the captain of your own ship.

One of the best pieces of advice Michelle ever received was this anonymous quote: *Other people's opinions of you are none of your business.*

PRIMAL WISDOM

Care about people's approval and you will always be their prisoner.
—LAO TZU (AS INTERPRETED BY STEPHEN MITCHELL)

Architect Language

Words have power at evoking emotions. Through our friend Mark England's program Procabulary, we discovered how our culture often communicates in conflict language rather than architect language. Conflict language destructs, and architect language constructs. Conflict language focuses on what you don't want, and architect language focuses on what you do want. We had our entire company take this course, and it made a profound difference in Michelle's leadership style, our business, and our personal lives, too. We think it could be useful to anyone working on emotional intelligence.

MARK ENGLAND SAYS . . .

Mark England is the founder of the Procabulary program, and a relationship and life coach. Procabulary focuses on how language use influences emotions and behaviors. Here's what Mark says about language:

> Most people use their language to inadvertently talk themselves out of opportunity, creating excessive problems and mountains of self-doubt. Very few people learn to get their words to work for them, but you can use language to stay focused, create opportunity, and build self-confidence. If you wish to change your reality, begin by changing your language.

Anyone familiar with how the subconscious mind works knows that what you focus on grows because it becomes the center of your attention. Let's say you decide you want to buy a red BMW. Suddenly, you see red BMWs everywhere. They were always there—you aren't magically calling red BMWs into your environment—but now you are noticing them, and that gives you more access to and knowledge about them.

People use conflict language all the time. Think about how we raise our children. We are always telling them what we don't want: *Don't do that, don't touch this, don't fight, don't argue, stop it right now!* This is conflict language. Architect language would be: *I would like you to get along today, love on your brother or sister, play together nicely.*

Think about how people argue. Conflict language uses guilt-inducing, conflict-generating words like *should* and *can't.* It points the finger and deals in black and white, with words like *always* and *never.* Architect language removes those words. Because it focuses on goals, it becomes a language of manifestation. It's a vastly different way to operate, to focus constantly on what you want and not what you don't want. It's like the number-one rule of improvisation in acting: Always say *yes.* Instead of *no* and *but*, it's *yes* and *and.* It's not, "No, you did it all wrong," or "I love you, *but* you have some serious issues." It's "I see what you are saying, *and* my perspective is a bit different" or "This is great work, *and* I would love to see you build on this part." Architect language builds people up instead of tearing them down, and it makes it easier for someone else to respond rather than react.

Unprocessed Trauma and How to Release It

In the case of serious trauma, these strategies may not be enough. Sometimes, you're not just offended by something. You're truly, deeply, emotionally harmed by something. What do you do about that?

We used to know. We are the only species that no longer uses our instinctual mechanisms for releasing trauma from our bodies. All living things can face trauma, and animals have ways to release it. When animals experience trauma, they throw themselves on the ground and shake and shiver. Remember that gazelle being chased by a lion? After the gazelle escapes, the first thing it does is throw itself on the ground and start shaking, to get rid of that trauma. It can look like an epileptic fit, but when it's over, the gazelle gets back up and goes back to its gazelle business. You can see dogs do this when they shake, as if they are shaking off energy. They will often do this after someone with high energy pets them (just watch!).

PRIMAL WISDOM

When the shake is truly valued and protected, it will keep the
spirit alive. Through shaking, the tight grip of totalizing ideology is
loosened. Shaking is a medicine to help prevent the hardening of
conceptual categories. It keeps our vessel open for the spirit to flow
through. As the Lakota medicine man Fools Crow put it, "We need
to be a hollow tube for the great spirit to pass through." Shaking
helps keep us a hollow tube and an empty vessel. And finally, it is
not only our bodies that have to be shaken; our words and meanings
must also shake. When the spirit moves through us, everything
will shake—our understandings, actions, and experiences.
—BRADFORD KEENEY

People also used to do this. Our ancestors threw themselves on the
ground, shaking and shivering to release trauma. There is a biochemical
explanation. When the brain perceives a severe threat, it triggers a cas-
cade of neurotransmitters and hormones that flood the system—stress hormones like adrenaline and cortisol pour into the bloodstream, as calming
hormones like serotonin and dopamine plummet. This causes a surge of
energy. When the threat is gone, the body has to get rid of all that leftover
adrenaline, and seizure-like shaking helps clear it so dopamine and serotonin can come back up to normal and the body can switch back out of
fight-or-flight and back into rest-and-digest.

People don't usually react like this anymore because of how it looks:
weak, scared, weird. We've had it shamed out of us, taught from childhood
to brush it off, man up, or suppress the release with sedatives. When a
child gets hurt physically or emotionally, the first thing we do is put our
hands on them, shush them, tell them to stop crying, tell them they're fine.
We fear they might be hurt, so we convince them they aren't. We try to
stop them from feeling their feelings because it's painful to watch a child
in pain, but this stops the child from going through the process of experiencing fear, pain, or grief. We pick them up and soothe it away, but this
teaches them that something is wrong with strong feelings and that they

need someone else to fix their trauma. This turns into learned helplessness and robs them of the opportunity to process the trauma themselves. As adults, that trauma simmers below the surface for years, or for a lifetime. We can't think of a better argument against helicopter parenting.

We believe unresolved trauma is largely responsible for the drastic rise in mental illness as well as the epidemic of violence we are currently experiencing worldwide, but especially in the US. It's controversial to say, but some people believe that chronic diseases like cancer, heart disease, and autoimmune diseases can be the result of suppressed emotional trauma in the body. Children in particular who repress trauma at a young age, especially when the trauma happened at the hands of a trusted adult, may develop severe mental illness later in life. Their physical bodies find ways to separate the conscious mind from the traumatic feelings, and the result can be extreme. (For a deep dive into the passing down of trauma through generations or even from past lives, check out *The Body Keeps the Score* by Bessel van der Kolk. To explore how disease can be traced back to stored trauma, check out the book *The MindBody Code* by Mario Martinez.)

PRIMAL WISDOM

The tissues possess an infallible memory for trauma. Everything is recorded in them.
—JEAN-PIERRE BARRAL AND ALAIN CROIBIER
(FROM THE BOOK *TRAUMA: AN OSTEOPATHIC APPROACH*)

Emotion Interventions

Physical experiences can cause emotional reactions, but the physical can also be a tool for healing the emotions. We've both experienced this first-hand. Until a few years ago, Michelle had never experienced real clinical anxiety, but after a severe mold exposure, she began to feel unusually anxious. It started when she felt nervous about doing routine phone calls. Day by day it got worse until she was having her assistant reschedule phone calls at the last minute because she couldn't bear the thought of doing them. Soon, she was unable to go to the grocery store or even leave the house. Finally one day, in the face of an important deadline she felt unable to meet, she couldn't stop crying. She was so overwhelmed and anxious that she felt like electricity was coursing through her body.

Keith called her doctor, who referred Michelle to a therapist in Austin who specializes in trauma and practices EMDR (eye movement desensitization and reprocessing, a type of bilateral eye movement or tapping therapy used for PTSD and other trauma, as well as anxiety). Within two sessions, all Michelle's anxiety symptoms were gone.

The therapist used knee tapping to disrupt the anxiety spiral to find the root of the problem. In Michelle's case, it turned out that her thyroid was damaged, and that was causing all the trouble—imbalanced hormones can really do a number on your mental state! She was finally able to get back into balance with thyroid medication (yes, sometimes, medication really does help), and she has never experienced anxiety that extreme again. Sometimes she feels it a little, but she learned coping strategies, like tapping, NLP, and meditation (see pages 147–148), to deal with it, and she has been able to keep it under control ever since. Without those initial interventions, she may never have gotten to the root of her anxiety.

Keith also experienced EMDR in therapy when he was struggling with some issues related to shutting down instead of feeling and processing his feelings. His therapist walked him back to a period in his youth when he had to deal with an unstable emotional situation. The therapist had him visualize everything he went through on a certain day—she asked what he felt, what he saw, what he smelled, what he heard, and Keith felt like he was right there in the situation. He could feel the disturbance in the emotional weather of his household.

After the therapist got him back into his childhood home, Keith said, "I can feel what's getting ready to happen." She asked what he was going to do and he said, "I'm going to get on my bike and get the fuck out of here right now!" When she brought him back out, Keith realized that he had been running (or riding, as the case may be) away from intense feelings about women since he was a kid—while also hypercompensating by trying to stir up trouble with men. Once he was able to recognize this, he could notice when he was doing it in his adult life, so he could work on reversing the knee-jerk response to flee (or fight).

Many trauma interventions are based on disrupting negative thought patterns that play like a looped song in the subconscious, and these can be quite effective, but most of these are not DIY interventions (we've mentioned when they are in the following list). We're not certified to tell you how to do any of these, but there are many different kinds of practitioners and techniques that can help. Here are some we've had success with. Find more information about them all on our Resources page at PrimalUprising .com/BookResources.

- **Tapping or EFT** (emotional freedom technique) uses systematic tapping with the fingers on different parts of the face and body to help interrupt negative thought spirals and reprogram emotional response. You can learn to do this yourself. We recommend the book, website, and app for *The Tapping Solution* by our friend Nick Ortner.

- **NLP** (neurolinguistic programming) uses the language of the mind to consistently achieve our specific and desired outcomes. It uses a form of self-hypnosis, timeline therapy, and other techniques to create and maintain desired emotional outcomes. We have both been trained to use it for our own emotional well-being.

- **EMDR** (eye movement desensitization and reprocessing) is described above. This type of psychotherapy is specifically designed for anxiety, PTSD, and traumatic memories.

- **Psychedelics,** such as MDMA, psilocybin, ketamine-assisted therapy, or other plant medicines administered by an experienced shaman work in similar ways to other trauma intervention treatments, by interrupting the repetitive thought patterns and introducing a broader perspective so people can break out of where they have been stuck. (We'll talk more about other uses for this therapy in the Spiritual Pillar section.)

- **Meditation** helps you work on being an observer of your thoughts and your emotions, feeling them, and letting them go. Michelle uses a technique where she visualizes sitting on a riverbank, watching her thoughts and feelings floating by. She can reach in and grab one and look at it, check it out, and feel what it feels like, but then she throws it back and lets it float away. Michelle finds this technique really helps her to be aware of her feelings without letting them trigger her.

DR. DAVID BERCELI SAYS . . .

A technique for relearning how to process trauma out of your body is TRE (tension and trauma releasing exercises). Our friend Dr. David Berceli is an expert in trauma intervention and conflict resolution. He created TRE to tap into our instinctual response to shake and shiver to release trauma. You can do TRE on your own for anxiety (see our Resources webpage at PrimalUprising.com/BookResources). For trauma, we recommend working with a practitioner. Here is what he says about TRE:

> The tremor mechanism in the human body appears to be an essential component of our self-regulatory system. This implies that all humans have access to this self-regulating human mechanism as a means of supporting self-care. TRE is about teaching this mechanism to others and guiding them to learn how to use this "new" body mechanism in a safe and effective manner to support self-care. [I believe] neurogenic tremors should be considered a fundamental human right just like the United Nations declared water, food, and sanitation as fundamental human rights.

Emotional Freedom

The Bigs are watching us all the time. They have us all pegged. They know what we like and dislike on social media. They know what we buy, what sites we visit, what groups we join, and they sell that information to whoever could profit from it. They have extensive digital dossiers on us (check out the compelling 2020 Netflix documentary *The Social Dilemma*). They know we don't want to believe or think about the uncomfortable opposing view, so they preach to the choir, get people riled up about the "other," and then they own us. The final remedy to this emotional control is simple: *Practice being uncomfortable.*

Listen to people you disagree with. Don't just wait to talk. Try to understand their perspective. You may come out of the conversation still passionately believing what you believe, but at least you experienced a little emotional discomfort. Physical discomfort builds physical resilience, and emotional discomfort builds emotional resilience. This can be especially challenging when someone else has strong convictions that disagree with yours, but what does it hurt to hear them? Convictions are emotionally charged opinions, not facts (although they can be based in facts, or perceived facts). They are neither right nor wrong. Nobody has the right to say that somebody else's convictions are right or wrong. What becomes right or wrong is the imposition of beliefs on someone else. Conflicts almost always stem from the imposition of values or perspectives, not the values or perspectives themselves. Recognizing that others have different values and perspectives is the beginning of understanding. You will know you have achieved emotional resilience when you can listen to passionate arguments you disagree with and maintain your equilibrium.

PRIMAL WISDOM

Your right to swing your arm leaves off where my
right not to have my nose struck begins.
—JOHN B. FINCH

Let's not be a nation of people spouting our opinions on the hill we are willing to die on, all the while stuffing our fingers into our ears yelling "*Lalalalala*" when somebody else tries to talk. Let's not be animals pressed into the corner, snarling and lashing out viciously at everyone we perceive to be attacking us. Let's not let them divide and conquer us.

If you can think and feel and communicate without being a bully, or a snowflake, and not be offended if someone calls you a bully or a snowflake, you are already winning. And always remember there is no such thing as certainty because as soon as you are certain, you're captive to somebody, somewhere. You're ripe for manipulation and control.

So question. Listen. Explore. Search. Know that you don't know what you don't know. And feel. Feel it all, own it all, take responsibility for it, even if it makes you throw yourself on the ground and shake. Release it all, shake it off, and get back to your life. Remember what it feels like to be a human again.

PRIMAL UPRISING LITMUS TEST

> Do you let yourself feel your feelings?
> What triggers you?
> Are you able to listen to emotionally charged convictions you don't agree with and respond rather than react?
> Do you take responsibility for your emotions and how you express them?

PART V
THE
SPIRITUAL
PILLAR

All differences in this world are of degree, and not of kind, because oneness is the secret of everything.

—Swami Vivekananda

11

FREE TO UNIFY

> As soon as you begin to take yourself seriously, and imagine that
> your virtues are important because they are yours, you become
> the prisoner of your own vanity and even your best works will
> blind and deceive you. Then, in order to defend yourself, you
> will see sins and faults everywhere in the actions of other men.
>
> —Thomas Merton

Spiritual wellness often gets lost in the shuffle of our busy and stressful lives. In practice, spirituality is about wonder, awe, and an exploration of consciousness. This is as essential for optimal health as good food, exercise, and stress management. In fact, as you'll see, spiritual health can make building health in the first three pillars easier and more natural.

Spirituality was woven into our ancient ancestors' lives. It was part of the everyday, not just a couple of hours at a service on the weekend. Nature was sacred, animals were sacred, the mysteries of the human body were sacred, and their lives were laced with ritual and reverence.

You don't have to be a churchgoer to find that space in your heart. It's already in there and you have access to it, even if you've never really focused on it before. To believe in nothing is to be empty, and to miss an important part of the human experience. True health can exist only when there is something bigger than ourselves to believe in.

The Benefits of Belief

Belief offers benefits that touch all the other pillars, and that's supported by a huge body of research. One comprehensive study took a bird's-eye view survey of all the high-quality scientific literature published between 1872 and 2010 (along with a few important studies published after) on spirituality, religion, and their influence on mental and physical health. The results were significant.[30]

First, the researchers looked at studies on how religion or spirituality helped people cope with illness (including blood disorders, cancer, cardiovascular disease, chronic pain, dental problems, diabetes, HIV/AIDS, irritable bowel syndrome, kidney disease, lupus, psychiatric illness, pulmonary disease, neurological disorders, and vision problems) and adverse life situations (such as bereavement, caregiver burdens, end-of-life issues, overall stress, natural disasters, war, and acts of terrorism). Almost across the board, those with religious or spiritual practices did better, recovered faster, and suffered less.

The study also showed significant positive relationships between religion/spirituality and well-being, happiness, hope, optimism, meaning and purpose, self-esteem, a sense of control over one's own life, and positive character. There was a significant inverse relationship between religion/spirituality and depression, anxiety, suicide, psychotic disorders like schizophrenia, bipolar disorder, substance abuse, social problems, and negative personality traits. The study author theorized that there are a couple of straightforward reasons why spirituality/religion is so beneficial for mental health:

1. Religion and spirituality generally provide more resources for stress management, counseling, a more optimistic worldview, and an underlying sense of benevolent support and trust that things will be okay.

2. Most religions have guidelines for how to live and treat other people, which can decrease stress and offer a framework for successful

living. People often aren't sure what to do, and having "rules" can help, whether they are the Ten Commandments, the yogic *yamas* and *niyamas,* or the five moral precepts of Buddhism. (These all have a lot of crossover, by the way.)

3. Most spiritual traditions emphasize loving others and serving as well as social gathering. These "prosocial behaviors" can reduce stress and create support networks. (We also know from other research that acts of kindness and helping others have positive mental health effects.[31])

The study also showed positive effects of religion and spirituality on lifestyle habits. People with a spiritual life engaged in less cigarette smoking and more exercise, and tended to have a better diet and healthier sexual behaviors.

To us, this is good evidence to support a more actively spiritual life, but that doesn't mean you have to run out and attend the next church service (that's your choice). There are many ways to cultivate spirituality. Religion may be your path, but you can also be spiritual without necessarily being religious.

PRIMAL WISDOM

Science is not only compatible with spirituality; it is a profound source of spirituality. When we recognize our place in an immensity of light-years and in the passage of ages, when we grasp the intricacy, beauty, and subtlety of life, then that soaring feeling, that sense of elation and humility combined, is surely spiritual. So are our emotions in the presence of great art or music or literature, or acts of exemplary selfless courage such as those of Mohandas [Mahatma] Gandhi or Martin Luther King Jr. The notion that science and spirituality are somehow mutually exclusive does a disservice to both.

—CARL SAGAN

Spiritual but Not Religious

You don't need to put a label on your spiritual life. While some of the research on the benefits of spirituality concentrates on particular religions, much of it is more all-encompassing. In fact, 25 percent of people in the US (ourselves among them) consider themselves "spiritual but not religious."[32]

To be spiritual means to believe in something greater than yourself, but also to see that greatness within you. How that works depends on how you want to express your spirituality—it might be through love, study, service, prayer, or ritual. Who you believe in also depends on you. It may be God or Goddess or nature or the universe. Maybe you don't really know what you believe, but you believe there's *something* out there because you've felt it. Even if you can't articulate it, engaging with it means you are acting as a spiritual being.

No matter what your spiritual life looks like right now, you can build on that base and get spiritually healthier. You can pray, meditate, read spiritual texts, meet with groups of people to discuss spiritual issues, ponder reality all by yourself, reach out and help others, look for the good, all in the service of keeping an open mind and your sense of wonder intact. You are a miracle, and so is this life. When you act as a spiritual being, you live that reality.

What we actually know is just a drop in the universal bucket. We have a lot more to learn about "life, the universe, and everything" (to quote *The Hitchhiker's Guide to the Galaxy*). We won't ever learn or understand it all in this lifetime, but there is no way to get around the fact that we were created somehow. We came from something beyond—we are literally composed of stardust. All you have to do is look around and think, *Okay, what are the odds that I would exist right here, right now, in this time and place, as this exact person?* You are a 300-million-to-one marvel. Awesome, indeed!

PAUL CHEK SAYS . . .

Riffing on an ancient quote, Paul Chek, the author and founder of the Chek Institute, says,

> God is a sphere whose circumference is nowhere and a center whose location is everywhere . . . If you know you are a center, then no matter what you put out into the world, guess where it has to come back to? You, because you are the center of the universe. Because you are a point of consciousness with self-reference. Because without you, there is no universe . . . no day, no night, no life, no nothing. You are the epicenter of everything . . . Meditate on that.

Look Within

The first aspect of spirituality, to us, is about exploring the depths (or heights) of our own consciousness. You don't have to agree with us on the details to agree with us on the big picture: that there is more to you than a body, a brain, and feelings, and that there is more to life than being born, living, and dying. We can't prove it, but we can feel it deep within.

Every morning, we both take some time to be alone with ourselves—for example, Keith likes to journal, Michelle likes to meditate or read scripture or something uplifting. Starting the day this way, instead of launching into emails and to-do lists the second your feet hit the floor, sets a more spiritual and satisfying tone to the day. As you look within, consider the ultimate question: *Who am I?* It's something to ask during prayer or meditation, and to ponder throughout your days. You can use the question to understand your own behavior, your thoughts, your experiences. It doesn't have to be organized. Just look within, during those quiet moments, and contend with what you find. Some of it may be full of light. Some of it may be full of darkness, but that's where the growth happens.

Once you begin to plumb those depths, you will discover how vast and limitless you are. We are all just one little point away from each other. That alone, we think, is enough to bring wonder to life. Who are you? You are all, and everyone. You are self, and you are other. You are the least of us and the greatest of us. You are a speck of dust and you have God within you. (At least, that's what we believe.)

Looking within can help you understand that only you are responsible for your happiness. No other person has control over whether or not you choose to be happy, but you do have to choose happiness. Instead of focusing on all the things you don't want (remember the discussion of architect language in chapter 10), which will get you more of what you don't want, focus on being fulfilled. Just as in meditation you can become the watcher of your thoughts, through introspection you can become the writer of your stories, using them as tools for your growth rather than dictators of your reality.

WHAT ABOUT SUFFERING?

We've had some interactions with people who are very spiritual and who have denounced the human body—the meat suit, if you will. They say the body is just baggage and this human experience is an illusion that has nothing to do with the much more real esoteric spiritual consciousness. To them, all the meaning is in the ether. But, as the Buddha said, "Only within our body, with its heart and mind, can bondage and suffering be found, and only there can we find true liberation."

We respect everyone's right to believe what they want, but to us, there is a reason why we're here, on Earth, in these bodies. Part of the human experience is to explore and discover that reason. Sure, it can feel at times like all of life is suffering; there is all manner of violence and turmoil in the world. How tempting to believe that none of it is really true! Yet spiritual wholeness is about finding the joy, delight, and lightness along with the pain and suffering. Light stands in high relief against darkness, and it is that interplay of light and dark, joy and sadness, euphoria and pain, that makes the whole experience worthwhile.

Spiritual Captivity

We think most people can probably admit that while religion has done many great things for many people, it also has its own dark side and its problematic elements. The Bigs have used religion throughout history to frighten, shame, guilt, and thereby control.

Every Big Religion has its punishment agenda: unless you act in certain ways, you'll go to hell or God will abandon you or you will accumulate bad karma or be sentenced to perpetual rebirths or whatever it is. They want you to bow to authority and do what they say, but true spirituality is spiritual freedom, not spiritual captivity. True spirituality seeks to empower you to look within to find truth, because that is where God is. You can find spiritual freedom within religion, but you can certainly find it beyond religion.

Do your spiritual beliefs and practices result in something positive for you, or something negative? For example, maybe for you, an all-powerful God is a comfort and you like knowing you are guided. Or, maybe that feels oppressive and you resonate more with the idea of the divinity within you that empowers you to guide your own life. Maybe your spiritual practices create joy, or maybe they create guilt. This is a clue to whether your practice is one of freedom or captivity.

It's always been our ethos to question and live in a place of uncertainty. We often go back to the Zen idea of a beginner's mind—one that is open, not rigid, and always ready to develop and change based on new information. We always try to see the world as if for the first time, look within as if for the first time, and let it all be new, every time. This is how to experience wonder. For us, that's where the juice of spirituality is, rather than in the rigid structure of a religion. But that's just us.

There is nothing we hold so tightly that it threatens our being—nothing we hold so tightly that we can't see it in a completely new way. We think spirituality should be an opportunity to become fully who you are, not molded into some preconceived notion of goodness. At the end of the day, doubt and questioning and fresh perspectives should strengthen belief, not weaken it. And this, ultimately, is how you make your faith resilient.

PRIMAL UPRISING LITMUS TEST

> Does this spiritual practice empower me, or am I handing over my power to someone/something else?
> Does this spiritual practice make me feel good, right, and strong, or does it make me feel weak, dependent, or guilty?
> At the gut level, does this spiritual practice make me feel expansive (good, free) or contracted (bad, captive)?
> Is this belief system strong enough that it can withstand doubt and questioning? Or is it such a delicate structure that it will collapse under any scrutiny?
> Does this spiritual practice expect/encourage an outward expression of my best self, or does it ask me to edit, limit, or repress an outward expression of my best self . . . or, worse, claim that I have no best self without intervention from outside myself?

12

BECOMING SPIRITUALLY RESILIENT

... When the [human] race sees its problem with clarity, it will act with wisdom, and train with care its Observers and Communicators. These will be men and women in whom the intuition has awakened at the behest of an urgent intellect; they will be people whose minds are so subordinated to the group good, and so free from all sense of separativeness, that their minds present no impediment to the contact with the world of reality and of inner truth. They will not necessarily be people who could be termed "religious" in the ordinary sense of that word, but they will be men of goodwill, of high mental calibre, with minds well stocked and equipped; they will be free from personal ambition and selfishness, animated by love of humanity, and by a desire to help the race. Such a man is a spiritual man.

—Alice Bailey, writer

To be truly spiritually resilient is to be able to withstand questions, including your own. The spiritually resilient person is not threatened by someone else's beliefs, and understands when it's right to evangelize and when it's more appropriate to take a step back and respect that others believe differently. The spiritually resilient person also understands that no earthly being or institution—not a religion, a guru, a priest, or a belief system—has all the answers. You don't have to imitate anyone else's spiritual path. Other people can inspire you, and their ideas can open your mind to new concepts and new perspectives, but you still need to go through the work to integrate those concepts and decide whether they feel true for you.

To hone that spiritual resilience, you can engage in specific spiritual practices to further open your mind to the mystical possibilities of the miraculous universe within you and outside you, always questioning, always putting your own beliefs to the test, but never being afraid to embrace what feels right.

Let's start with one of the most basic but powerful spiritual practices anyone can do: journaling.

Journaling

Journaling may seem simple, but it can be transformative because it can open a direct line to your subconscious. One way we like to use it is as a mode for asking our higher selves for guidance. To do this, think about what your questions are, or what is happening in your life that you aren't sure how to handle. When you feel ready, start writing. Don't think about what you write, just let it flow, and don't edit. Free-write, and the answers will frequently come through. Journaling works because your higher self already has all the answers. You just need to remember them, and journaling is a way to get there. Michelle likes to do this every morning, as part of her gratitude practice. She begins by writing down all the things she is grateful for that morning, and then the wisdom begins pouring out of her pen.

A dream journal can be another useful tool. Your dreams are filled with meaning and symbolism. While you sleep, your body detoxes and your mind processes, consolidating memories and making sense of your experiences. It also works on your problems. Dreams can help you understand what's bothering you, offer solutions you hadn't thought of, and guide your decision-making. You may need to do some interpreting— there are some standard symbols you can learn about from dream interpretation guides, but you don't really need them if you employ your intuition and your journal. To journal your dreams, write them down first thing in the morning, before you look at your phone or do anything else. Dreams fade quickly! Sometimes, you'll get the meaning right away. Sometimes you won't see it until you come back to your journal later and read what you wrote.

Meditation for Spiritual Growth

Meditation is a mental tool but it can also move you into a spiritual terrain where you can better perceive your vastness and infinite nature. Meditation can help you to face things you believe about yourself, the world, and your experiences that may only be stories. It brings perspective to the petty worries of daily life. You may contend with trauma and encounter strong emotions like grief as well as positive ones like joy and ecstasy, and meditation can help you to feel them, process them, and then let them go so they don't haunt you anymore.

The actual nuts and bolts of meditation will vary from person to person (refer to pages 119 and 164–166 for guidance about different techniques). Don't be locked into the idea that meditation means sitting in the lotus pose and chanting. It can be that, for sure. Or, it can be getting lost in a wood-working project or lifting weights, as it is for Keith. It can happen while utilizing a sensory deprivation tank, a Lucid Light, or an Opus sensory immersion bed. To some, meditation can be a religious experience, a communion with God. For others, it is more an exploration of the infinite depths of the self. (Or it can be both, since God lives within the infinite depth of the self.) Whatever you need from meditation, it can be there for you.

IS MEDITATION SACRILEGIOUS?

A common misconception about meditation (and yoga and other practices that originated with religious traditions outside the traditional Judeo-Christian framework) is that it is evil or opens the door for evil things to enter your mind. This is simply untrue (unless you choose to believe it—perception creates reality, after all; but ask yourself, who told you that story?). Where you go in meditative contemplation depends on you, but since God is within you and you are a child of God and part of God via the holy spirit (or however your belief system describes the holy aspect of the self), you are always protected and safe. It's just you and God in there, and meditation can be a way to commune with that higher power.

If you're really not comfortable meditating, or don't see it the way we do, you might prefer prayer, which isn't much different. Prayer reaches out to something higher, but also goes deep within to feel the answers and guidance. As long as you are taking this quiet time for spiritual contemplation, reflection, and exploration, you will be working on your spiritual growth. It doesn't matter what you call it.

Moving Meditation

Most people meditate while sitting, but for others, like Keith, sitting still is torture. Keith wrestled with this concept for a long time. He felt guilty that he wasn't sitting in the lotus position chanting "Om." A few years ago, he was sharing his frustration with a friend who asked, "Why does meditation have to look like that? You're a physical being and a kinesthetic learner. Why do you think you have to sit in the lotus position? You can move. If it gets you into that meditative state, it doesn't matter what you're doing." It was a revelation for Keith, that he could use movement as meditation and the gym as his "church."

Moving meditation can be done while walking, running, doing yoga, or lifting weights. It's similar to being in flow state—utter absorption and focus on an external activity, as opposed utter absorption and focus on the internal activity of meditation. Melding the two is a powerful example of the sum being greater than its parts. As long as you can be quiet and go inward, your body can be doing anything.

Weightlifting is Keith's form of prayer. It takes him out of his everyday mode of thinking and into a more spiritual place. Keith has the skill level to lift properly without hurting himself, so he doesn't need to pay such close attention to what he is doing. (It's important to practice moving meditation only with a movement you can do without thinking too much about it.) That's why most people choose walking. For some, walking in nature is the most spiritual thing they can do. If it lifts you up and makes your spirit soar, then it is a spiritual practice.

MEDITATE ACCORDING TO YOUR LEARNING STYLE

We all learn in different ways and operate in different modes. There are many ways people learn, and many combinations. For example, some people are visual learners who need to see something to learn it. Some people are auditory learners who learn better if they hear the explanation. Some, like Michelle, are audiovisual learners, who need to see and hear at the same time to best take in the information. Some are logical, mathematical learners who do best with numbers and scientific principles. Some like Keith are physical or kinesthetic learners who need to move and touch and participate to understand. Social learners learn best around other people. (These are just a few of the many learning styles.)

You probably have an intuition about what your own learning style or styles might be, and this can guide you toward the type of meditation that you might enjoy most. Here are some examples:

> **Visual learners** often prefer visualizations for meditation— picturing all the details of a scene, whether they guide themselves through it or listen to someone else guiding them through it. Meditations that begin with "Picture yourself on a sunny beach" or "Picture yourself in a peaceful forest" are easy for visual learners, who may also enjoy gazing at a candle or doing mandala meditation (gazing at an intricate circular design as a point of focus—the center represents the state of one-pointed consciousness).

> **Auditory learners** may prefer guided meditations that walk them through relaxation techniques to get them into a

more meditative state, like meditations that begin: "First, relax your toes, then your ankles . . ." Auditory learners also tend to like mantra meditation, where the sound of a repeated word ("om" or any other simple word or phrase) helps them get into a meditative state, and/or meditating to music. They may find meditating in silence difficult.

> **Mathematical learners** are good at counting techniques, like counting breaths or counting backward. They may also enjoy meditating on sacred geometry designs or natural forms, like the center of a flower or a cross-section of a snail shell, or repeating mantras while manually working along a strings of mala beads, with one bead per mantra repetition.

> **Physical/kinesthetic learners** like Keith usually prefer some form of moving meditation. They can get into a meditative state more easily if they are doing something. Walking meditation is great for physical learners, but for those who can sit still, holding mala beads can help with concentration because it gives fidgety hands something to do.

> **Social learners** may do best taking a meditation class or meditating with a group, such as with a prayer group or at a Zen center. They also tend to like doing meditation retreats better than those who prefer more solitary meditative practices.

Sound Healing

The human body has an energy frequency, and when we hear sound, our frequency can adjust to it. This can result in profound emotional release and healing. Sound can also launch you into a meditative state more quickly by exposing you to the high vibrations associated with positive energy, love, and spiritual understanding.

Every day of Paleo f(x) starts with an invocation and sound healing. Sound healers come on stage, chant, and play tuning forks, singing bowls, bells, and chimes. They have the most amazing voices and they know how to use them and their instruments to push out negative energy and put people into a more open, spiritual state of mind, setting a tone of grace and ease for the day.

The first time we did this, our audiovisual team was backstage helping get everything ready. They asked Michelle what was going on and she said, "Oh boys, you're getting ready to go to church!" The sound healer had some people lying on the stage to feel the vibration. Once everyone was situated, she began singing. Everyone around her rode those waves of sound. The AV guys stopped what they were doing. They were blown away. These guys have done AV for Google and other big corporations all over the world, even for the Pope, and they had never experienced anything like her voice. These grown men were standing backstage, overcome with emotion.

As Michelle sat in the front row listening, she could feel her emotions releasing and she started to cry a little, too. She was about to do an interview, and she saw the woman who was going to be interviewing her—a radio personality from Dallas—step into the auditorium. Michelle got up and quietly led her to her dressing room backstage to do the interview. As soon as Michelle looked her in the eyes, the woman burst into tears. She said, "I'm so sorry! I have no idea why I'm crying!"

"It's the sound healing," Michelle explained.

"Really, I'm just so sorry," she said. "I don't know what's wrong with me."

Michelle repeated, "It's the sound healing. There's nothing wrong with you. That's what's supposed to happen. Whenever you need to release something, the sound helps you." It was interesting to see someone who had never experienced sound healing before have such a profound release. We all hold things that will ultimately make us sick if we don't let them go, and sound healing is a powerful way to stir them up and move them out.

Sound healing may seem "woo" but many Paleo f(x) speakers who are scientists have come up to us after the sound healing to tell us that they have never felt this kind of high-vibration frequency before. Just because we don't fully understand how it works doesn't mean there isn't real power behind it. Earth itself has a vibration (called the Schumann Resonance, or the "heartbeat of Mother Earth"[33]), and the closer to that we get, the more in tune with our environment we feel. It's like medicine from the planet.

Drum circles can be another kind of sound healing. Michael Harner, an anthropologist and founder of the Foundation for Shamanic Studies, has explored shamanic traditions in different cultures around the world, and he discovered that drumming was a primary vehicle for entering into a shamanic experience in many different cultures.[34]

We highly recommend sound therapy for a spiritual tune-up. Michelle is doing this by taking shamanic voice lessons, to open up all her vocal resonators, which has helped her channel through singing. See the resources to find out more about this.

Ritual—Any Ritual

One of the pushbacks we often hear against religion is the idea that it is full of empty rituals, but we believe all rituals can be spiritually beneficial. Anything can be a ritual. When our son Kleat played baseball, his team always had a pregame ritual, whether at home or away, that began exactly one hour before first pitch: a perfectly timed choreography of warm-up exercises leading into more complex drills. They played specific music that got the kids to speed up throwing a baseball to each other. The ritual built their confidence and psyched out the other team. It got everybody's head into the game, and their team ended up going to the Babe Ruth World Series.

When you do a ritual regularly, you train your central nervous system to expect that repetition. The ritual itself isn't the mystical part. It's a tool to prepare the body and mind for a spiritual experience. People who fear rituals that don't coincide with their beliefs are misunderstanding their purpose. Here are some rituals that might work for you:

- **Traditional religious services.** These include many rituals, depending on the tradition. Revisit participation in a religious tradition from your past, or try a completely new one, if you're so inspired.

- **Yoga.** Yoga prepares the body for meditation by exercising and limbering up. The ancient yogis would often sit for many hours at a time, and yoga was a way to get their bodies ready for this. A specific series of poses you always do before meditation can help you feel less restless and more able to focus.

- **Affirmations/devotionals.** Saying or thinking affirmations before you start your day is a ritual that puts your mind in a more positive, open place. Spending some time each morning and/or night reading a devotional or a spiritual text can send you into your day or night with a calmer, more compassionate perspective.

- **Breathwork.** Practicing different breathing techniques, or the yogic practice of *pranayama*, can calm the central nervous system and center the mind, whether you use it prior to meditation or before doing something that is stressful, like giving a speech or taking a test.

- **Communing with nature.** Going outside, walking through a natural area, or sitting under a tree and being mindful of the natural world around can be a sacred ritual to put you back in touch with Earth and the real world around you. This is a great ritual to do when you've been on your computer or phone too much.

- **Seasonal/special occasion rituals.** Whatever you celebrate, making rituals around those celebrations can make them feel more sacred and meaningful, whether it's welcoming the new season, celebrating any holiday, marking the passage of time (birthdays, the new year), or creating (or resurrecting) your own personal or cultural rituals around the events that mean the most to you. These kinds of rituals add flavor and soul to life.

Plant Medicine for Spiritual Growth

We can't talk about the Spiritual Pillar without going a little deeper into plant medicine, since that has been such an important and revelatory experience for us personally. Plant medicine ceremonies involve taking psychoactive substances for the purposes of enhancing consciousness exploration. There are many plant medicines, as common as marijuana and as exotic as ayahuasca. Several years ago, we were called to this practice, and it has had a more profound influence on our spiritual lives than anything we've ever done—it has transformed us both and added great value to our lives.

Michelle first got interested in plant medicine after Brittani's death. She had heard stories and discovered through research that plant medicine journeys can allow contact with people from the other side, and she so desperately wanted to communicate with Brittani that she decided to try it. The plants helped her work through her grief in powerful ways.

You don't necessarily need the plants to achieve the kind of spiritual breakthroughs we have experienced using them—you can open new neural pathways and expand your consciousness through other practices such as meditation, but it's a way to fast-track the process. You can do a lifetime's worth of spiritual work in this truncated period of time. The plants have taught us many things, including how to fulfill our own needs with love and compassion for ourselves and others, rather than for selfish reasons; how to see ourselves as expressions of divinity; and how to vault into states of higher consciousness. When we come out of ceremony, we almost always feel profound love, true gratitude, and unity. To us, this is what makes it all worthwhile. All the shit we have to go through in this human experience is justified because of the love.

The shaman we worked with initially always told us, "You don't need this substance to get to where you're going. It's just a shortcut." Once you know that other realm exists, you can get there any time you want to. That reminded us that the power wasn't so much in the plants as within us. The plants only helped us become aware of it, and aware of what is possible.

Most of the benefits of plant medicine happen during the integration afterward. The ceremony opens the door, but the work is going through the door. The facilitator's job doesn't end when the weekend is over. A good facilitator can help you with the integration piece, guiding you through that process of incorporating what you learned into your life.

But again, like everything else, there is a shadow side to plant medicine. It can be a boost or it can become a crutch, when people rely on it and think they can't progress without it. People with addiction issues may not be good candidates for plant medicine ceremonies. If you are using drugs to escape your life rather than to step fully into it, you may be abusing these substances. If you have a history or family history of drug abuse, plant medicine may not be for you. If you have any doubt, hesitation, or fear in your mind, plant medicine is probably not for you. Some people simply won't ever be called to it. We would never push this on anyone. It is a calling, and only you can decide if you want to go there.

If you think the plants might be calling to you, we urge you to do your research and learn as much about what you want to explore as you can before engaging with it. A retreat under the guidance of a practiced and reputable shaman is the best way to begin. This isn't something to do on your own, and it's not recreational or "for fun." Consider who will take you through the journey. Vet them, whether they are shamans or facilitators. Is the shaman/facilitator looking to empower you, or keep you in perpetual need of them? It's the same for any guide. A good facilitator will never promise you something, like enlightenment or any concrete result. They cannot know what you will experience. They can only promise to keep you safe and offer a secure setting. Only the plants know what you need, and it may not be what you want. There has to be an element of surrender in it, and you must be prepared for that. One of the things the plants have taught us is that control is an illusion.

It's also important to recognize that just because a substance works for one person doesn't mean it will work or be good for someone else. Cannabis (marijuana) is a good example. Some of our friends love it, and it has been a great teacher for them, but it gives Michelle anxiety. You may not know if something will work well for you unless you try it. If you do, stay in tune with how it makes you feel. Pay attention to the way your body, mind, emotions, and spirit react. That's more important information for you than what anyone else says "should" happen. (And by the way, as with any medication, never operate a motor vehicle or heavy machinery when using any psychoactive substance.)

But Aren't These Illegal Drugs?

The legality of plant medicine varies by location and situation. You can do an ayahuasca ceremony legally in a church ceremony, as well as in some Native American religious settings (and in some other countries, but do your research before signing up for that—there are scams). You can use cannabis in certain states, but other things like LSD, psilocybin, ketamine, and MDMA (not all plants, but all used for consciousness expansion) aren't legal in most states. They may be soon—for example, hallucinogens are being intensely studied for psychiatric use, as treatments for depression among other things, and psilocybin is gaining legal ground—but we are supportive of anyone who doesn't want to do anything illegal.

However, we argue with the notion that anyone else should tell us what we can and can't do if we have done our due diligence and we don't put ourselves or others in (potential) harm's way. We believe that all should have the choice to use this therapy. Right now, those who do try plant medicine often face legal and moral judgment. We've experienced this from our own family and friends surrounding the use of these medicines, but we believe and hope this will change, as the understanding of spiritual and therapeutic tools expands.

DR. MOLLY MALOOF SAYS . . .

Dr. Molly Maloof is a biohacker and concierge doctor who uses plant medicine with her patients and follows the legal developments surrounding these promising therapies. She sees a new era of legality and use coming in the very near future:

The FDA has granted both psilocybin, the active ingredient in "magic mushrooms," and MDMA the title of "Breakthrough

Therapy" for their roles in the treatment of depression and PTSD. Breakthrough Therapy Designation (BTD) is given to investigational drugs for serious or life-threatening conditions. To be eligible for this designation, the medicines must show a particularly high effect size and offer substantially greater clinical benefits than existing options. We are entering a new era of psychedelics that will enable the careful and safe prescribing of these treatments to treat conditions plaguing humankind.

What Do You Live For?

The final piece of the Spiritual Pillar is purpose, and we believe everyone can explore it through spiritual pursuits, whatever they may be. What gives your life meaning? What makes your spirit soar? Why were you put on Earth? To serve others? Create beauty? Spread wisdom? How will you do that? We believe we are all here to serve in some capacity, to teach, and also to learn. For us, this has been through Paleo f(x). What will it be for you?

Whatever it is, it may change throughout your life, but think about what it is today, and let that purpose guide your decisions, both large and small. Let it be your North Star, and you will always know what direction you are going. To help you figure it out, let these questions be prompts for your contemplation:

- What are you good at? What are your talents?
- What do other people say you are good at?
- What do people come to you for advice about?
- What nonmaterial things do you desire in your life?
- What do you do that makes time dissolve and puts you in a flow state?
- What do you think the world needs most?
- Who or what do you feel most passionate about helping?
- What moves you? What brings you to tears with emotion?

- Imagine yourself ten years from now. What do you hope you will be doing?
- What is your dream?
- What are five ways you could use your talents and passions to make life on Earth better in some way?

We hope you will continue your own spiritual explorations. This can be the most rewarding pillar to strengthen if you really commit to the journey. Whatever way you choose, remember to be discerning.

PRIMAL UPRISING LITMUS TEST

> Am I using this practice to explore or to escape?
> Am I using this practice to do spiritual work, or just for pleasure?
> Is the person guiding me looking to empower me, or keep me in need of them?
> Do I use this practice as a tool to expand my own consciousness, or do I feel like I can't have a spiritual experience without it?
> Does this practice bring me closer to my life purpose, or is it a distraction from my life purpose?

PART VI
THE
FINANCIAL
PILLAR

Money is only a tool. It will take you wherever you wish, but it will not replace you as the driver.

—Ayn Rand

13

FREE TO GROW RICH

A wise man should have money in his head, but not in his heart.
—Jonathan Swift

There are few things about life in this world more complicated and fraught with false beliefs as money. Ever since humans invented the concept of trading a symbol for goods and services, we've mixed up money with power, worth, meaning, success, and love. We call it "the root of all evil" and the "solution to all problems," but money is neither of those things. The Bible actually says that the *love of money* is the root of all evil, rather than money itself (1 Timothy 6:10), and that gets closer to the problem. Money is not something to love or hate. Money is just energy. You can generate it in the service of whatever it is you choose. You can use it for good or for evil, but that's no reflection of money itself, just as the gasoline in your car's gas tank has nothing to do with where you choose to drive your car. Understanding this changed our relationship with money, and if you struggle with the financial pillar, we hope it can change yours, too.

LOGAN STOUT SAYS . . .

Our friend Logan Stout is a bestselling author, speaker, and entrepreneur, and we agree wholeheartedly with his take on money. Logan says,

> That money is "evil" is one of the most disempowering, crippling, and controlling of all limiting beliefs. Money is simply energy; the more you have, the more good works you can do with that energy. Money doesn't "make you" any way whatsoever. Money is just an amplifier of your current personality. Are you a whole, connected, giving, and loving person now? Think of all the good you could do with millions worth of "energy" to fuel your good works.

Energy is a resource, and without resources, life becomes stressful and insecure. That's why having money (energy) can alleviate some of the stress of worrying about survival and provide the means to pursue personal optimization. Money can facilitate freedom to do what you want, go where you want, and pursue your dreams. It's not the only way to have those things, but it's a useful tool. So why all the negativity placed on money? Why do some people disdain it or the people who have it, experience guilt about having it or not having it, feel squeamish about wanting it or earning it, or think they're inferior for not having enough? And on the other side, why all the obsession, greed, desire, self-aggrandizement, and feelings of superiority about having more of it than the next guy? Why are our ideas of money so skewed?

It can be hard to separate our culture's money values from our own, but in reality, beyond what we decide it is, money doesn't really exist. It's a made-up concept. It's bartering with a symbol. The Bigs have determined that money has value and have drilled that into our minds so that we believe it and accept it. We go along with the status quo idea that those who have more are better, and there is something wrong with those who have less. Or, we blame money itself for our problems with it.

But the energy you give money is the energy it returns to you. If you can separate it from the stories the Bigs tell you about it and step back from their efforts to manipulate you with those stories, you may see that *you* get to decide how you feel about money. What kind of energy do you give it? Greed energy, generosity energy, love energy, or fear energy? Do you give money energy that will bring you more of it, or that pushes money away? It's your decision. You can use the energy of money to get healthier and freer, or you can let others use and control you with the energy of money.

HEALTH IS WEALTH

Medical bills and insurance costs have financially devastated millions. Consider Detroit. The city had to declare bankruptcy, and one of the major contributing factors was that the city and county workforces were so unhealthy that they could not afford their rising health insurance costs.[35] Detroit was the canary in the coal mine. We believe we will see more and more of this kind of collapse if we don't become aware of the essential link between health and money. When we lose our health, we risk losing our financial security, and wrong as that is, the best way to guard against this potential disaster is by preserving health—which you can do by bolstering all the other pillars.

We've both made *and* lost a lot of money over the course of our lives. We've both struggled with negative feelings about money and felt victimized by it, especially when we lost everything in the 2008 housing crash. When we started Paleo f(x), we realized that we would not survive without money, so we set a positive intention: to make people healthier and stronger, to help them live richer, more valuable lives, and to set them free from the constraints of a dehumanizing system. If we could make money educating others about how to be truly healthy and empowered, then we believed money would come to us. And it did.

But money mindsets can be deeply embedded, and that often starts in childhood. Many of us have had childhood experiences that formed our feelings about money. To get to the root of your money memories and money attitudes, you may have to go back in time.

IF MONEY WERE YOUR LOVER . . .

Our friend Jolie Dawn, who is now a money coach, wasn't always as money-savvy as she is now. When she was young, her father took his own life because of his financial situation. She blamed money for her father's death and grew up hating money because of what she perceived it "did to" her father.

It took her a long time to realize that money didn't do anything to anyone. Her turning point came when her mentor asked her, "If money were your lover, would it want to have sex with you?" That completely changed her perspective. Was she attracting money as she might attract a potential lover, or was she repelling money the way she might repel someone she wanted nothing to do with? We attract and repel money much the same way we attract and repel people. It's all about the energy we put out. Now, she is an expert and advises other people about how to manage their money issues.

Money Memories

Because of the power our culture gives money, early money experiences can carve deep grooves in the subconscious mind, causing people to think and act around money in ways they don't fully understand. Because we are involved in groups with so many other entrepreneurs, we've heard these stories many times, and we have our own.

Keith grew up with the attitude that he wasn't one of those lucky people who got to have money. He came from a working-class family, and they instilled in him that if you wanted more money, you worked overtime. Rich people got that way by screwing other people over. That mindset was drilled into Keith for his entire childhood and young adulthood.

Keith learned to be a survivor. Nobody could work harder or longer than he did. The idea that abundance is everywhere and you just have to focus on it for it to come to you was never his reality. It wasn't until, as an adult, when he began to crave freedom in his life, that he realized the only way to be truly free was to have financial freedom. When he began working for Big Pharma, suddenly he had a lot of money, but he never felt financially secure or happy with the work. He wanted to make a difference in the world, but he couldn't square that with wanting to make money. It took a lot of work for him to recognize that money is energy. Only then was he able to get comfortable with entrepreneurship.

Michelle's story is more personal, and for anyone who might be sensitive, we are officially giving you a **content warning about sexual abuse** now. Michelle debated telling this story here, but decided it would be worth sharing because of how it shaped her conception, not just of money but of her own worth (which is so often intimately tied up with money).

When she was four and a half years old, Michelle was essentially trafficked by her babysitter. Michelle remembers her babysitter taking her out to the stairs of her apartment building and telling her to wait there. The babysitter said that if Michelle left the stairs, she would be in trouble. Then the babysitter went into her apartment, leaving Michelle alone.

A man who had been lingering nearby behind a shed staring at Michelle approached Michelle as soon as the babysitter was gone. He took Michelle into the laundry room and raped her on top of a washing machine. She passed out, and when she awoke, the man told her that she would be in big trouble if she told anyone what happened. She immediately remembered that she wasn't supposed to leave the stairs, so she thought it must be her fault. Michelle had an empty jar with her that she used to collect flowers, rocks, and bugs. The man opened the jar, threw a quarter in, and gave it back to her. She didn't tell anybody what happened to her. She didn't want to get in trouble again.

About two years ago, Michelle was working through this experience in a plant medicine ceremony. When she got to the part about the quarter in the jar, her facilitator stopped her. She said, "Michelle, wait . . . what is your relationship with money?" This was a seminal moment for Michelle because she realized that she had been paid for the rape . . . and as a four-year-old, she was worth exactly twenty-five cents.

She has since been able to heal from that trauma, but she had never before considered how it had influenced her relationship with money. Michelle always had the feeling she didn't deserve money, and as soon as she earned it, she let it slip away. She could never hold on to it for very long. After that session, Michelle was finally able to put money back in its rightful place as a tool—as energy only—and not as some measure of her worth, or something she did or did not deserve.

Michelle's feelings about money were also influenced by her father leaving the family when she was two years old. Her father became very wealthy, while she, her sister, and her mother constantly struggled. Her mother had some of the same issues—she couldn't hold on to money, either. If she earned five dollars, she spent ten dollars. Her mother was always battling her father to take care of his own children financially. They all felt, each in their own way, that he didn't consider them worthy of his money, let alone his time and attention, and Michelle spent her childhood in an environment of scarcity and lack. Like Keith, she thought abundance was something that happened to other people but not her and her family.

As a culture, it often seems we put far more value on money than we do on people, but humans are priceless. There is no amount of money that could ever equal a person, but many of us have had to go through a long dance to come to that realization.

Here are some other things we have realized about money along the way. These are basic concepts about money that anyone working to strengthen their financial pillar might consider:

- You are either attracting or repelling money, depending on how you think about it and use it.
- Money is not responsible for what is wrong in your life. Only you are responsible for your life. Blaming money repels money.
- When you focus on what you don't have, you repel money.
- When you focus on gratitude for what you have, you will feel like you live in abundance and you will attract money.
- There is nothing wrong with desiring things, unless the desire becomes so strong that you don't appreciate what you already have.

- There is nothing inherently inferior, or inherently noble, about being poor, and there is nothing inherently superior, or inherently immoral, about being rich. Anyone can be noble, and anyone can live immorally. It's about you, not the money.
- There is a profound difference between being technically broke and being (feeling) poor. Broke is a moment in time. Poor is an attitude and a lifestyle.
- Having a good life is a choice that has nothing to do with money.

Does Money Buy Happiness?

If money is energy, and we need energy for life, doesn't it make a kind of sense that money could buy happiness? People have studied this question, attempting to discover some magic number that buys happiness.

One of the most publicized of these research efforts was a 2010 study from Princeton showing that people who make less than $75,000 per year feel more stress in life, but that anything above that level did not increase happiness.[36]

Two years later, in 2012, Skandia International came out with a report putting that sweet spot at $161,000.[37] Raising the stakes higher, *Town & Country* magazine reported in 2017, based on their research, that the amount of money it would take to feel fully free to pursue your passions, support causes you believe in, live wherever you want, give your kids a top-notch education, and generally never have to worry about money, was about $100 million![38] Quite a leap from that $75K in less than a decade!

Now, $75,000 may seem like a lot or a little to you, and $100 million may seem pie-in-the-sky or possibly doable. The truth of course is that there is no one number because it all depends on what you want out of life and how good you are at using money's energy. Some billionaires keep trying to make more because they never feel they have enough. Others just want to continue to pursue their passions, and money happens to flow from that. Some live extravagantly and some live modestly. Warren Buffett is a billionaire, but he reportedly said that he would be perfectly happy living on $100,000 per year. He lives in the same house he has lived in for half a century. Meanwhile, many people win the lottery and blow all their winnings in less than a year.

There are no rules and there is no certainty when it comes to money. It can help bring you the things you want, and it could lower (or increase) your stress, but whether you are happy is a choice that has nothing to do with money. If you think you need more money to be happy, then maybe you should look inside yourself for the real cause of your unhappiness. There are plenty of miserable rich people. Our dear friends Tah and Kole Whitty (we work on personal development with them) say that the only difference between someone who has money and someone who doesn't is that one person is crying on marble and the other is crying on linoleum. We are all still subject to the human condition, and money can't hold and comfort you in your sadness.

Consumerism

Money is one thing, but what about all the stuff you can buy with it? Isn't that why most people want money, to get more stuff? We are a consumerist culture, and people love to go shopping and associate themselves with their possessions, whether it's a fancy car or designer clothes or something else. How many Amazon packages have been delivered to your doorstep this year? How much stuff is in your house that you never use? You spent life energy on each one of those things—you worked when you might have been doing something you would rather do, all to earn money to be able to buy those things (sometimes on impulse) you don't really need or want.

Big Business is genius at convincing people that they need, or at least want, those shiny objects that promise a better life. People actually get a dopamine hit to the brain when they press that "buy" button or open that package, and they can get addicted. When the high wears off, they go right back to their shopping apps to get another hit. It's that little devil constantly whispering in our ear that if only we had this or that, we would finally be happy, or beautiful, or cool, or popular, or a success, or that everyone will envy us and want to be us.

Why do we care if anybody wants to be us? The Bigs have convinced us that this has value. They've schemed to keep us in financial captivity. If we are obsessed with money and possessions, we are distracted, and Big Business gets richer. If they keep feeding us two-day delivery packages and streaming services and apps, we may not notice that we are less and less rich in those things that have real value. We keep falling for it because it feels so good in the moment. Even when we know, logically, that financial freedom is more desirable than possessions, we keep buying things. Consumerism has stolen our life-force energy. We may try to use money for good, but we do so in a system set on using money as a weapon.

A materialistic lifestyle will never propel us forward as a culture. Remember when Ronald Reagan lowered interest rates and told everybody to "Go for it"? Remember after 9/11 when George W. Bush said, "We can't let the terrorists achieve the objective of frightening our nation to the point where . . . people don't shop"?[39]

We all have a choice. Each one of us can decide if we are victims of the financial system, or if we will instead choose to take control. We can choose to be grateful for and satisfied with all that we have now, and we can work to be free of the attitudes and actions that keep us captives. We can strive to make our lives better and more in keeping with our values—and we can remember that a good life doesn't have to involve a single online purchase or trip to the mall, let alone an expensive car or a big house.

What are your values? What really makes you happy? Your first answer might not be your real answer. Think about how you will feel on your deathbed. Did anybody ever say, "I wish I would have had more stuff"? Probably not. What most people do say is that they wish they would have spent more time with the people they love, traveled more, enjoyed their lives more, let themselves be happier, and felt more comfortable with being who they are. Money makes some of those things easier, but is that what you are spending it on?

Abundance Is a Choice

It can be hard, especially if you are living in scarcity, to really believe that abundance is a choice. You may see other people who have it so much easier and think that you can't ever escape your situation. We've both been there, and we both also acknowledge and recognize that the world does not offer a level playing field. There will always be inequality. There will always be somebody who has more or has it easier. There may be trauma in your past, or beliefs so deeply ingrained that you have to work really hard to uproot them. You may feel stuck, trapped by poverty, inequality, and a system that keeps you down. You can feel like it's unfair to be at the bottom of the barrel, and it is. Some people seem to have all the luck, in what happens to them, or just because of where or how they were born. Situations are obstacles and indeed, some of us face mighty ones.

But for every mired-in-poverty-and-scarcity story, there is an example of someone who overcame their situation to become happy and wealthy. Just as with feelings (or happiness), you cannot always control the situation, but you can always control how you respond to that situation.

Keith remembers when playing football how his team could sometimes make every move perfectly, execute every play, and still get beaten because the other team was bigger or faster or maybe just luckier. It wasn't the team's choice to win or lose, but it was always Keith's choice how he would handle the loss, and what he would do next to keep getting better. Just because he wasn't going to become the world's best football player didn't mean he would stop trying to get a little better every day and do a little better in the next game. Most of us will never be billionaires, and some of us may never rise above the poverty line, but as long as you have the mindset that it is someone else's fault and you are stuck and a victim, you won't escape that cage you are in. The way to move forward is to take responsibility and make choices that point you in the direction you want to go. Step by step, choice by choice, anyone can alter their course.

Even though we believe in the importance of finding happiness now and feeling gratitude for what you have, we also believe it's okay to want more. We can all think of things we would like to improve about our lives and things we want to add to our lives. It's good to have goals and desires. It's what keeps humans moving forward in their lives.

What's dysfunctional is that "I can't" attitude on one end, and that "never enough" attitude on the other. Those are both just stories. Who told you that you can't? Who told you that you don't have enough? You can work toward more from a place of worthiness and abundance, rather than from a place of unworthiness and scarcity.

KRISSTINA WISE SAYS . . .

Our friend and money coach Krisstina Wise has helped us completely reframe our ideas about money. We think her course should be taught in every high school. Here is some of her wisdom:

Freedom is the essence of all living things. Nothing yearns to be caged; there are no poems written about longing for leash and chains. And yet we—either consciously or unconsciously—sabotage our freedom with poor health and financial burden. While it's true that money can't buy happiness (it's only energy, of course), what it can do is leverage opportunity. Opportunity paves the way for sovereignty. And only from a place of sovereignty can you then choose (demand?) freedom. Every sovereign being has the opportunity to ask: *Is it worth my freedom? This purchase, that habit, this relationship . . . is it moving me closer to the freedom I desire? Or is it another bar in the cage?* On the flip side, everyone can ask: *How much money is enough? Am I working at something I love? Or am I indentured in service of things that I really don't need or want?* "Is it worth my freedom?" isn't just a theoretical question. It just might be the question of a life well lived.

Just as any good health habit can be small but accumulate over time, every good financial choice can be small but will accumulate over time, both in resources and in shifts in your own mindset. Every time you don't buy something you don't really need, you'll get better at making that kind of choice. Every time you put some money into your savings account, you'll get better at making that kind of choice. Every time you decide *not* to trade your life energy for something that will impede your freedom, you'll get better at making that kind of choice.

You can live a life of abundance, no matter what has happened to you in the past and no matter how you grew up thinking about money. You can break that cycle and build a strong financial pillar that will support the happiness you deserve.

PRIMAL UPRISING LITMUS TEST

> ❯ Do you want something because you really want it as a part of your life, or do you just want the thrill of buying it in the moment? (To help you answer this, imagine how you will feel two weeks after buying that thing.)
> ❯ Do you wish you had more money so you could buy more things, or do you wish you had more money so you could pursue your life's work?
> ❯ Who told you that you don't have enough, or are not worth having more? Why did you believe it?

14

BECOMING FINANCIALLY RESILIENT

Successful people make money. It's not that people who make money become successful, but that successful people attract money.

—Wayne Dyer

Financial resilience grows out of experience and perspective. It is a product of gratitude for what you have and conscious awareness of what you trade your life energy for, as well as an awareness of when the system is trying to control how you spend your money and where you put your attention. How do you begin doing all that? Let's start with minimalism—not living without the things you really love and need, but trimming away what is holding you back, so that your life better reflects what you want it to be, without all the baggage.

Mindful Minimalism

We prefer minimalism that allows for spending our money energy on things that bring more meaning to our lives, rather than wasting it on the accumulation of possessions or on costs that we can avoid by staying healthy, strong, and sharp. This doesn't mean getting rid of all your possessions.

There are many different ways and systems for practicing minimalism, but what they all have in common is discernment about possessions, drilling down on what you really need, and backing away from a consumerist mindset that uses buying things as an emotional pacifier.

You can start practicing minimalism very simply, by questioning what you buy before you hit that buy button. Every purchase has the ability to chip away at your freedom, and through that lens, we can better determine whether the purchase is worth it or not. This is a powerful way to be mindful about the real value of material things.

We each like to practice minimalism in somewhat different ways. Michelle likes the KonMari Method popularized by Marie Kondo in her book *The Life-Changing Magic of Tidying Up*. This is an easy and inspiring way to begin decluttering what you already own, category by category, starting with the easiest and ending with the most difficult to declutter objectively: clothes, books, papers, miscellaneous items, and sentimental items. It's a very satisfying process, and Michelle really enjoys going through each category and getting rid of what we hold on to for no good reason—or condensing what matters into a more manageable form. After Brittani died, we had so many things of hers—more than it made sense to keep. To help, Michelle took pictures of Brittani's things and made an album. Then she donated the items to Goodwill, so someone else could use and enjoy them. This was a solution to the difficult problem of getting rid of sentimental items, and Michelle often looks through that album. It's an easier and lighter way to remember.

Keith approaches minimalism more philosophically. He's a fan of Joshua Fields Millburn and Ryan Nicodemus, "The Minimalists," who promote minimalism specifically as a tool for finding freedom (by now, you have probably figured out that freedom is Keith's thing). On their website, they say that minimalism can help you find "Freedom from fear. Freedom from worry. Freedom from overwhelm. Freedom from guilt. Freedom from depression. Freedom from the trappings of the consumer culture we've built our lives around. Real freedom."[40] They agree there is nothing wrong with possessions if they add value to your life, but if they compromise your health, relationships, or personal growth, they are keeping you captive. Check out their documentary, podcast, books, blog, or their free e-book: *16 Rules for Living with Less.*

Keith also likes the concept of vagabonding, which is a minimalist way of life Rolf Potts describes in his book *Vagabonding: An Uncommon Guide to the Art of Long-Term World Travel,* and also as described in Tim Ferriss's *The 4 Hour Workweek.* These books sealed the deal for Keith when he was considering bailing on corporate America. *Vagabonding* is about life on the road, which requires minimizing possessions and prioritizing experiences over things—that is the key to the minimalist ideal, that material objects can act as numbing agents, like watching TV or binge eating candy. More philosophically, we are here to experience, not to have. Anybody who dreams about traveling will get caught up (obsessed?) with this concept and the steps to make travel happen *now* rather than waiting for some unsure future to do what you've always wanted to do.

A place to start is to ask yourself: *What is the minimum I need to live a fulfilling life?* Or, alternatively, *What do I have now that is keeping me from living a fulfilling life?* Having things isn't the same as being materialistic. We aren't championing scarcity. In fact, moving away from a materialistic life can actually make you wealthier because you won't throw your money away on things that don't matter anymore. Materialism is a prison and minimalism is freedom.

Spending is just one part of minimalism. Earning is the other part. People are so often trapped in jobs that keep them from doing what they really want to do in life, just because they have to keep paying for all the stuff they have—the expensive mortgage, the big car payment, all the subscriptions and services and things and spaces to put all the things. We need the energy of money to live, and making a lot of it in the service of the right, the good, and the free is a noble cause. If you can live on less and keep earning, that's great. Or, maybe you will live on less so you don't have to keep earning so much, or so that you can take a break and reassess what you really want to be doing with your life. When you earn money doing something you are passionate about, and you use the money energy you earn to fuel your passions and talents, then you will have a healthy, robust financial pillar.

At the heart of all of this is making peace with money. We hope you will think deeply about your relationship with money and where you may be stuck, giving it more (or less) power than it deserves. Remember that money is only energy, and how you spend it is your most immediate access to democracy. It's a "vote" for whatever product or service you buy, and that is reason enough, we believe, to spend money only on what you truly believe in. The Bigs are experts at siphoning this energy from you, but once you understand this, you can keep that energy for yourself and use it in the service of your own freedom and happiness.

Financial Freedom

According to a 2019 consumer debt study by the credit reporting company Experian, consumer debt in the US is $14.1 trillion, and the average personal debt load for each American is $90,460.[41] These debts include credit cards, mortgage loans, student loans, personal loans, and lines of credit. When you owe money, you aren't free, and although many will tell you that being in debt is just part of the American way, we say: Then let's change the American way!

We shouldn't have to be beholden to the Bigs just because we can't stop buying stuff, but most of us are. The only way out of the financial prison that is debt is to pay it off. Where are you now, and where do you want to be? Can you scale back and pay down your debts aggressively, or are you able to do only a little at a time? Every little bit helps. It's like changing anything else—your diet, your fitness, or any other bad habit. Step by step, consistently over time, you can make big changes.

The first thing we did to tackle our debt was to decide we were no longer willing to play this game. Next, we connected with our friend and wealth coach Krisstina Wise (quoted earlier), who helps people understand how to organize their money and create wealth, to learn more about how we could improve our financial health. We got better at assessing what we really needed and refreshing our priorities. We began to practice different aspects of minimalism. We became more aware of the influence of advertising. We went through all our regular payments and figured out which ones we could happily discontinue.

Now we are taking it to the next level, looking to buy land outside the city limits and work on living off the grid to extricate ourselves as much as possible from the whole financial system. Meanwhile, we continue to prioritize our health above all else, so we can minimize the chances of incurring huge medical debts down the line. We keep working on optimizing all our pillars so we can be as strong and independent as possible. We're making good progress. You can, too.

MONEY BASICS

Most people don't really understand how money works. Why isn't every high school student taught about debt, interest, taxes, and investing, or fractional reserve banking and how money can be created out of thin air?

The Bigs benefit when you don't know how money works, but the information is out there and you can learn it if you choose. The more you understand about money, the more savvy you will be in how you use it. Do your own research, or check our Resources page at PrimalUprising.com/BookResources for some of our favorite sources of sound financial information. There's a lot to learn, and some of it will probably surprise you—it sure surprised us!

Becoming Soulpreneurs

When you are your own boss, you get to make the rules and you aren't under anybody's thumb. But in a way, you are under the thumb of the company you create, if you want to be able to make enough money to live. When we first became entrepreneurs, there were many times when we dipped into our personal bank accounts to keep it going. Then one day, we had the opportunity to meet Darren Hardy. At the time, he was the editor of *Success* magazine (now he is a *New York Times* bestselling author, speaker, and advisor). He's one of the most influential leaders in the self-development and business world.

We were talking to Darren about our business, this whole Paleo f(x) conference we'd dreamed up, and he asked us: "Is it successful?"

We hemmed and hawed a bit, explaining that it was fundamentally successful but that we didn't really care about money, as long as it breaks even, because it's our mission, the legacy for our daughter, and all of that. Our first impulse was to emphasize that *because* it was a good cause, we *did not* care about the money.

He said, "Can I tell you something, and can you just be open to it and listen to me?"

"Sure."

He said it was great that we were mission-motivated rather than money-motivated, but that if we chose to turn Paleo f(x) into a profitable enterprise, we could build a bigger bullhorn. Making more money meant touching more people and changing more lives. But, Darren said, we would have to get over our "ick factor" around money, and if we couldn't do that, the fact that we weren't reaching the large numbers of people we wanted to reach would be squarely on us. Did we want to be the impediment to making more people healthy?

That discussion was a light-bulb moment for us. It helped us understand that making money wasn't a bad thing, especially when it meant helping more people than we could just breaking even. We saw that there was no more noble or better place to make money than in a pursuit that could change lives and get peoples' health back on track. Then we thought of the word: soulpreneur. We weren't entrepreneurs. We were soulpreneurs!

Paleo f(x) became about aligning the money-making side of our lives with the purpose and service part of our lives. Some people are entrepreneurs just to make money—it doesn't matter what widget they are selling today, next week, next quarter, as long as it's profitable. A soulpreneur doesn't operate that way. Instead, they make money for the greater good. When we made that switch, the money followed. We developed a mastermind group called Soulpreneur f(x) around this idea and quickly discovered how many others had the same problematic relationship with entrepreneurship. Like us, they responded enthusiastically to the idea of soulpreneurship.

From then on, our key performance indicators gauging what success looked like became very different. We weren't focusing on the money beyond watching expenses, and instead paid attention to how many new people we could bring into the Paleo f(x) sphere every year. That's when Paleo f(x) started making money, and growing faster than ever before.

We now envision our business as a mighty oak tree that requires tremendous resources to stay alive, more so than any of the surrounding trees or greenery. In return, it provides a vastly greater value in the way of shade, habitat, and beauty.

If you are already an entrepreneur, or want to become one, we highly recommend getting training so you can avoid some of the beginner mistakes that we made. Mastermind groups like our Health Entrepreneur f(x) are good midtier experiences. Multilevel marketing businesses can be a great entry point to start learning about owning your own business. Another way to get started is by "flipping" things, whether something big like houses or small things you buy, fix, and sell. However, there really is no fail-safe, entry-level school other than possibly apprenticeship, and the all-important school of hard knocks. Don't let that stop you. Go out and do what you were meant to do, and learn as you go.

No matter how you start, we definitely recommend going the soulpreneurship route. There is nothing more gratifying than making money in the service of the greater good by doing something you are passionate about. We are now hooked into a huge network of other soulpreneurs (whether they call themselves that or not), and our lives look completely different than they did ten years ago.

There will always be obstacles and financial bumps in the road, but when you are a soulpreneur, you don't just throw in the towel. You adapt (like when we had to move Paleo f(x) online during the coronavirus pandemic!). Remember, that's what resilience is all about. The most financially resilient businesses are the ones that can adapt to changing times, and the times are always changing. We keep working to make a difference and we will always have our mission, along with the faith that when we work to make the world better, the money will come.

PRIMAL UPRISING LITMUS TEST

> Do you understand your financial situation, or would you rather not know?
> Is your debt mostly from things you truly want (like a home you love), or because of things you can't remember you bought?
> Is your business aligned with your purpose?
> Is money a net stress or a net positive in your life? If it's a net stress, what is the first thing you can do to begin changing that?
> Are you making enough money to reach enough people?
> Is that thing you want worth the equivalent hours of work you would put in to earn that amount of money? Is it worth trading your time and life energy to have it?

PART VII
THE RELATIONAL PILLAR

Love is the vital essence that pervades and permeates, from the center to the circumference, the graduating circles of all thought and action. Love is the talisman of human weal and woe—the open sesame to every soul.

—Elizabeth Cady Stanton

15

FREE TO CONNECT

Love much. Earth has enough of bitter in it.

—Ella Wheeler Wilcox

So far, the pillars have been mostly focused on the self, but the last two pillars are just as important when it comes to wholeness, wellness, and resilience. These are the pillars that deal with our relationships: with family and romantic partners in this section, and with community, tribe, or "soul families," as we call them, in the next section of this book.

We are social by nature, and we cannot ever be fully whole or fully healthy in isolation. We need each other, but not everyone has healthy relationships. Let's explore why, and what we can do about it to achieve relational health.

Family Connection

You love them, you hate them, you didn't choose them, but you are (mostly) stuck with them. Or are you? Over the course of human history, the structure of what people call a "family" has changed quite a bit (although how, exactly, is a fraught area of anthropology and sociology!). If we could go back in time and take a look at how our distant ancestors lived, we would see scenarios as diverse as ancient diets were, and we are no better off trying to imitate the family structure of any particular ancient (or modern) culture than we are trying to eat like an Inuit or a Hadza. What we do know, however, from contemporary research, is that human connection has a profound positive influence on health if it is supportive, loving, and companionable. One study demonstrated that low levels of social interaction were as harmful as smoking fifteen cigarettes, or alcoholism; more harmful than never exercising; and twice as harmful as having obesity![42]

Today we have options and that means we could look to many different kinds of models as we seek a functional and satisfying family structure. One model that was once common to many cultures was the multigenerational family, and we think that's worth consideration. Can you imagine living in the same house with your children, parents, and grandparents? For most of us, with our busy lives, demanding jobs, and wealth, it's unimaginable. We need to work to afford modern life, which means outsourcing both childcare and elder care. For our ancestors, that was rarely an option, but for us, it's considered the norm. Once our kids can take care of themselves, they move on to their own households and that's just the way it is.

This modern way isn't all bad. We've gained freedom from these changes in the family structure and, honestly, we get it. We like our privacy, and while we love them, we wouldn't want to live with our parents at this point in our lives, when our kids are finally (mostly) out of the house. On the other hand, we do see that we've lost something by relinquishing those many years of physical proximity with other generations. We don't always know our kids as well as we would if we were always home with them, and we have devalued the older generations in our culture. We no longer prioritize their wisdom, knowledge of the past, and experience, so we don't get to learn from it.

But we have options. Maybe you like the way it works for your family, and maybe you don't. If you don't, what if you changed it? What might work for you? Would it be more functional for you if, instead of sending your children to daycare, you could have your grandparents or parents be with your children while you're at work? For many families, that's not an option. Grandparents often have much more active, independent lives than they once did and may not *want* to take care of children. In other cases, they may not be physically capable of childcare. But what if they can and want to do it? That could be a valuable upgrade for your family, including for your parents and your children, both emotionally and financially.

Let's go further. Would it be better to go back to having a multigenerational household? For some people it might be. When you all live together, duties like childcare, cooking, cleaning, and earning money can be shared, so one or two people don't have to take on that entire burden, or pay to outsource it. But for many families, this wouldn't work either. There are too many other things we all want to do, and we may not want to share our space. Only you can know what's best for your family, but what we hope you won't do is limit your options because of what is expected or most common. If it would work for you and your family to live in a multi-generational household, why not do it? It's nobody else's business. And if that sounds like pure torture? Lucky for you, it's probably not necessary and you can live your life the way you want to live it, as far away from your family as you need to be.

When Keith's kids were born, he and his first wife were very young and beyond broke. For them, it was most feasible for Keith's wife to stay home with the kids and for Keith to work, and that's what she wanted to do. Other parents wouldn't be happy doing this—they want to have careers and they know that someone else could do a great job taking care of their children. Other parents have no choice. They may need two incomes, or they may be single parents who are the only source of income. None of these ways are right or wrong. Children benefit from having happy, fulfilled parents who know they are working to support and guide their children, whether that means a parent is home all day or whether kids have other caretakers. The impulse to care for your family is ancient, but the way you do it can be very modern. No guilt! We do what we can. It's the same for aging or infirm parents and grandparents—maybe it works to have them at home with you, and maybe it doesn't.

The Dysfunctional Family

Family structure aside, what about family dynamics? Of course, you know there are as many different kinds of family dynamics as there are people. No family is perfect and every family has its quirks and issues, but what if yours is truly dysfunctional? How do you build a healthy relational pillar when, in your life, family equals suffering?

Some families can become toxic and emotionally harmful, either from what people in the family do, or because of what they don't do. In Michelle's case, the dysfunction came from having an absent father. Michelle's parents divorced when she was young, and she spent much of her life trying to have a relationship with her father. She used to quip that their relationship was off-again/off-again, but it wasn't really a joke to her. She was the middle-child peacemaker of the family, so she was always trying to repair the rift, and the repeated rejections were painful.

Michelle will never forget the Thanksgiving day when she was about 10 years old. The family was visiting an aunt in Texas, about an hour away from where her father lived. Michelle asked her mother if she could call her dad and ask to see him. Michelle didn't know that, at the time, her mother was taking her father to court for child support and insurance claims (he was wealthy and they were living below the poverty line). She and her sister Susan got on the line together and when he answered, Michelle was so excited! She said, "Hi Daddy! It's Michelle and Susan!"

He answered, "I don't have any daughters named Michelle or Susan," and hung up on them.

Michelle and Susan were shattered. Their mother did everything in her power to compensate for her daughters' pain during that holiday season, and Michelle still thinks about how it must have felt for her mother to see her little daughters' devastated faces.

But Michelle persisted. A few years later, she asked her father why she always had to call him and he never called her. He called her a prima donna, then said it was because he didn't want to hear her mother's voice. It wasn't until Brittani died and Michelle reached out to their father that she found any resolution. Michelle's father hadn't seen Brittani since she was two and a half. When Michelle called him, she could hear in his voice that he was assuming she was going to want something from him. Michelle broke the terrible news: "I don't know if you care, but I thought you should know that Brittani died."

Everything changed at that moment. Michelle could hear the regret and pain in her father's voice. He said, "I can't believe I never fixed this." He hadn't seen her in over twenty years, and it was too late. He asked Michelle if he could come to Brittani's memorial service. She said yes because she knew that's what Brittani would have wanted.

We tell this story to show you that dysfunctional families can heal, at least to a point. However, they don't always, and that's okay. There is a point at which we can handle the pain and forgive, but if you aren't at that point, it may be better to keep your distance. Healing is hard, and some people will never master it, or choose it. Forgiveness is harder, but that is where the balm for the pain exists.

Whether the solution is to separate or to resolve (or first one, then the other), a healthy relational pillar is built from the knowledge that healthy relationships aren't about what anyone did to you, or didn't do for you. They are only about *you* and how you choose to respond to the actions of those who may have hurt you. As with so many other parts of life and health, we are all 100 percent responsible (as adults) for how we decide to live, who we decide to interact with, and whether we decide to be happy. There are no *shoulds* about what to do, or whether to reconcile. How you contend with the relationship in your own head is the only work.

Love Connection

Let's move on to love relationships. We are both passionate about how to navigate and optimize our marriage. How do you keep romance alive? How do you grow together instead of apart? And in our case, how do you work together without killing each other? To illustrate how difficult this can be, we'll start by telling you about how our own marriage almost didn't survive.

Couples who work together can find it difficult to separate the personal relationship from the working relationship, and there is nothing romantic about working long hours together every day to keep a company afloat. After we both decided to go into business for ourselves, together, we took on a lot. We jumped at new opportunities and before we knew it, we had multiple businesses—several gyms, the supplement company, and then, of course, Paleo f(x). The stress was overwhelming, we weren't always sure of our roles, and we were with each other all the time. Many factors added to the stress, some of which we've already told you about. Michelle struggled with how to be a leader. She also struggled with the constant assumption that Keith and other male partners had always assumed the men were in charge, when Michelle was actually running things. This made Michelle resentful. Keith struggled to find his role, and the workload was crushing for both of us. It all came to a head when (as we mentioned before), Michelle suffered from a severe mold exposure. Losing her mental sharpness and excellent memory had always been one of her greatest fears, but after the mold exposure and everything else, she couldn't keep thoughts in her head. She felt scattered all the time.

Her response was to lash out at Keith. She took her anger and frustration out on him, and as he naturally withdrew from her, she became increasingly resentful and fearful. We had made an agreement, when we decided to get married, that our relationship would always be intimate, close, passionate, and romantic, but that was fading fast. Michelle felt that Keith wasn't doing his part. She thought she was doing all the work to keep the relationship afloat, but of course blaming him wasn't inspiring him to step up. Instead, Keith's reaction was to shut down, so our communication got worse and worse until one day, Keith exploded and poured out everything he'd been holding back in a flood of anger. Until that moment, Michelle was able to maintain the illusion that everything was stable because Keith never got angry. When he finally did get angry, we both realized that our marriage really was on the rocks and that we might not make it. We had started as friends and we thought that would always be our bedrock. Everything was built upon that, so what happened? We went into the marriage knowing it was meant to be, and it terrified us that we might have been wrong.

A lot of things could have happened at the peak of our marital dysfunction. Some relationships end at this point—some are probably meant to end. But we weren't ready for that, so we decided we had to try to save our marriage.

We began to work on our marriage. We sought counseling from multiple sources, including our Human Design coach and through more traditional counseling. Key for us was recognizing that we were each responsible for our own part in the relationship. Neither of us owed the other anything. No, our marital life was the result of our own choices. That made each of us focus on ourselves instead of what the other person was or wasn't doing. We also realized that if we didn't put some boundaries on our business, our relationship wouldn't survive and then neither would Paleo f(x)—meaning Brittani's legacy wouldn't survive. Our entire business was built around the seven pillars of health, yet we weren't honoring them ourselves. We felt like such hypocrites! We'd forgotten our priorities.

The first thing we did was make a decision as a company to walk the talk. How could we build a foundation of health if we worked until midnight every night and made our employees do the same? The entire company agreed that we would no longer work at night, except during the run-up to the show because that was crunch time. It wasn't easy for any of us to learn to turn off work, but gradually we all adjusted to putting work aside after 6:00 p.m.

Then we turned to our own relationship. We recognized that our marriage was a mutual co-creation. It wasn't something happening to us. We created it the way it was, so we could create something different. Because of Human Design, we were able to discover that each of us had certain intrinsic qualities we couldn't change, and we had to accept those in each other if we wanted to make it. We also discovered all the areas where we *could* compromise and come to more mutually beneficial decisions. We took all the tools we could get. We learned everything we could. We became more creative participants in redesigning our marriage, and today, we're stronger than we ever were before we went through that crisis.

Let's Talk About Sex

Fixing our marriage also meant fixing our sex life. We won't go into those personal details, except to say that when communication and intimacy break down in a relationship, it's common for sex to taper off. Restoring an intimate, consensual, sexual relationship is an important part of fixing a marriage or other romantic partnership.

Even though it's so important for relational (and physical and emotional) health, people are often afraid to discuss sex with each other. We find all kinds of reasons to make sex embarrassing, uncomfortable, taboo, or shameful. Why? Sex is one of the most basic primal instincts we have, both for reproduction and for pleasure.

When we are ashamed of sex, it can be used to control us. When we think there is something wrong with us for how we think or feel about sex, we cannot achieve sexual health. The truth is that there is nothing wrong with anybody's desires or preferences. Nothing. There are certain kinds of desires that, if acted upon, would hurt someone, and that's wrong. But there is nothing wrong with fantasy. Those who act out harmful desires (such as assaulting someone) have often been hurt themselves, or they are not wholly integrated and are unable to acknowledge and control their own shadow side. (Sex is probably the most charged and susceptible area in which the shadow side expresses itself.) Sexual health is about acknowledging and taking responsibility for your sexual life, and that often begins with talking about it.

In the US and some other countries, many families don't openly discuss it with children and prepare them for what's going to happen to them, even though we all know that as soon as you make something taboo, adolescents are going to go straight for it. If we don't want our kids experimenting with sex, we need to discuss it openly so there's no curiosity or mystery to go find out what it is—and of course, healthy experimentation is a growth experience for some adolescents, depending on their maturity and the circumstances. What's not healthy is to shut down the conversation— or never having it in the first place!

Michelle's parents had Michelle when they were young and unmarried, and Michelle's mother never told Michelle anything about sex—Michelle didn't even know what sex was. The only "sex education" Michelle received was in fifth grade when the teacher explained that girls get periods. When her best friend got pregnant in high school, Michelle asked her, "How can you be pregnant if you aren't married?"

"Duh, the normal way," her friend said.

"What do you mean?" Michelle asked. She didn't think it was possible to have a baby if you weren't married.

"Are you kidding me?" her friend said.

"No, I'm not kidding. What do you mean?"

Michelle ran home to ask her mother, and her mother told her some horrifying story about having sex. It sounded disgusting. "I'm never doing that," she said. (She never equated any of this to what happened to her when she was sexually abused as a child.) Yet, Michelle ultimately ended up perpetuating the same cycle, having her first child out of wedlock, and so did her sister and her brother.

As adults, even if we weren't brought up to feel comfortable talking about sex, we can learn to do it. A few years ago, neither of us would have ever dared to actually talk about our sexual desires to each other, but we've learned how to be completely honest and open about it now, and it has transformed our intimacy. Don't get us wrong, it wasn't easy. There were some very uncomfortable moments as we worked through the emotional obstacles to talking about sex, but this is something couples can work on together, and it starts with a simple conversation. (We'll tell you about how we approached this in a therapy session, in the next chapter.)

The shame, guilt, and discomfort surrounding sex is exactly why we have discussions about sex at Paleo f(x). We want to bring that out into the open so it doesn't get so repressed that it comes out as perversion. We need to normalize it in the context of loving, consensual relationships. We are wired for desire, and if we can't talk openly about it in our intimate relationships, we can't achieve as deep a level of intimacy as might be possible. When you can be open and honest about your desires, it becomes a healthy part of sexual play with the person you love, making sex more exciting and fun.

The bottom line is that sex is *natural,* not wrong, not shameful, not perverted. We are meant to enjoy it, and it is such a pleasurable boon to intimacy that it is worth the effort to fix the broken parts, when you are ready.

CHRISTOPHER RYAN SAYS . . .

There is a wide range of normal, in sex and otherwise. Our friend Chris Ryan, author of *Sex at Dawn* and *Civilized to Death*, has studied human behaviors and has come to this conclusion:

> From savoring saliva beer or cow blood milkshakes to wearing socks with sandals, there is little doubt that people are willing to think, feel, wear, do, and believe pretty much anything if their society assures them it's normal.

PRIMAL UPRISING LITMUS TEST

> Do you make an effort to understand the family members in younger and older generations, so you can learn from them and they can learn from you?
> Are you happy with your family structure? Could it be better?
> Do you try to control other people or do you focus on controlling yourself?
> Do you think it is someone else's job to make you happy, or do you make yourself happy?
> Can you talk openly to your partner about sex, or is this difficult?

16

BUILDING RESILIENT RELATIONSHIPS

Human relationships are not fixed in their orbits like the planets—
they're more like galaxies, changing all the time, exploding into
light for years, then dying away.

—May Sarton

To have resilient relationships is to have relationships—whether familial or romantic, whether parent, child, sister, brother, cousin, friend, spouse, or lover—that are strengthened rather than destroyed by adversity. It is to transcend the idea that "you owe me this" or "I owe you that" and understand that you are solely responsible for your part in that relationship. To believe anybody owes you anything assumes that you need something you can't get on your own, and that somehow, miraculously, that other person has what will finally make you whole. What a burden to put on someone else!

With that in mind, this chapter is about how to think more deeply about your own role and responsibility in relationships, and put those self-discoveries into practice to strengthen your own self-concept and help you become more adaptable and compassionate. Relationships (especially romantic ones, but also in many cases relationships with family and friends) are not about partial people becoming whole. They're about whole people choosing to do life together. If you want to be in resilient and fulfilling relationships, you first have to become resilient and fulfilled yourself.

Radical Honesty

People hide from each other. We hide who we really are, even from the people we love the most, and often without realizing it, because what if the people we love won't love us, knowing who we really are? We even hide from ourselves, afraid we won't love *ourselves* if we fully admit to everything we are, from the best to the worst.

But that's exactly what stands in the way of true intimacy. Not only do each of us have to accept responsibility for who we are, but to have a fully healthy relationship, we need to show who we really are to our partner—and to fully see who are partner is, when they show themselves to us. This may sound scary and radical, and it is, but it's also the path to a radically amazing relationship.

In therapy, we both learned that one of the reasons we hid from each other was to protect each other. It took realizing that we didn't need to protect each other from who we were to stay married. It was the opposite: we had to *stop* protecting each other from who we were to stay married. In one of our therapy sessions, we participated in a game-changing exercise that helped us to step into radical honesty. We each had to write on a board everything we wanted out of our relationship. Then we had to tell each other everything we felt was problematic in the relationship, and when one of us was talking, the other one had to listen without interrupting.

Michelle remembers the torture of listening to forty-five straight minutes of Keith telling her the most uncomfortable things she'd ever had to hear about how her behaviors made Keith feel. She wasn't allowed to say anything or rebut anything, but this forced her to really hear Keith and recognize how much misunderstanding there was between her intention and his perception of what he received from her. She kept wanting to say, "Yeah but, yeah but." On top of that, our facilitator, Tah Whitty, kept telling Keith, "Don't hold back, get to the nasty stuff, let's go."

After that, Michelle had ten minutes to take responsibility for every-thing she had done. Not how Keith felt—that was his responsibility—but for all the things she had actually done, even when she didn't want to admit she'd done them. No justifying, no excuses, just taking responsibility. That was hard.

Then the tables were turned. Keith had to listen to everything Michelle felt about what he had done, and then he had to take responsibility for his actions and choices.

The next step was to tell each other exactly what we needed from the relationship. This was harder. We're so conditioned to soften our words because we know how it might sound or make the other person feel. We're conditioned to protect each other, at the expense of honesty, but the facilitators made us drill down to the core of what was true for us and say it. It was especially hard for Keith to actually express out loud what he needed. He remembers thinking, *C'mon, do this, she doesn't need your protection, stop protecting her, just tell her who you are! Be honest! If you're not honest, she doesn't really have you anyway. Say something!* He had always prided himself on speaking his truth, but when it came to baring his soul, the words wouldn't come for a good forty-five minutes. Then it was Michelle's turn.

Finally, we had to say to each other, "I'm not responsible for how you feel. I'm only responsible for how I feel. This is what I want, and what-ever your feelings about it are, that's not my problem. I love you. I care about you."

This was some of the hardest work we've ever done, but it changed how we saw each other, and it changed how we viewed the relationship. There is Michelle, and there is Keith, and then there is the relationship. Instead of putting the relationship first and protecting each other from any so-called truths we think might hurt the relationship, we were forced to admit who we were, decide what we wanted, express it fully to the other, and then choose whether to respect each other as individuals. This is what actually strengthens relationships. When you are radically honest, you let the person who loves you share your burdens and your fantasies with complete acceptance of them and of you, while you each take full responsibility for your own feelings and needs. Your relationship will hit a completely different level when you're no longer protecting or expecting.

Everything we wanted, needed, and put on the other person was really on us all along. Each of us can control only ourselves. We can choose to give or receive, talk it out or be silent, tell the truth or lie, stay together or end the relationship, but nobody else is responsible for anybody else's happiness. Recognizing and especially *internalizing* this truth completely changed our partnership dynamic. Could it change yours?

PRIMAL WISDOM

The cave you fear to enter holds the treasure you seek.
—JOSEPH CAMPBELL

No Judgment

The last part of the work we did was to stop judging. Radical honesty requires radical trust, and that's scary because we all fear judgment. Being radically honest about who you are has another side: being radically accepting of who your partner is. That doesn't mean you won't get angry or irritated with them sometimes. We get upset and frustrated with each other all the time. The difference is that you accept who they are anyway, annoying parts included, and you don't judge them for it. Love and respect are the defaults. Who they are is 100 percent their business, just as who you are is 100 percent your business. To be in a relationship is to choose to accept this. It's an amazing, magical thing to know that someone in the world accepts you completely and unconditionally for exactly who you are in every way, and doing that for someone else is a great gift.

To summarize it all, deep intimate loving relationships really require only three things:

1. Radical honesty about who you are.
2. Total responsibility for what you do and how you feel. Nobody made you do or feel anything—you chose it.
3. Total acceptance without judgment of who your partner is.

Saying "only three things" makes it sound easy, and of course it's not. Doing these three things is one of the hardest jobs we have as humans, but there is nothing better than the relationship that will emerge when you master them.

How Much Do You Want It?

All of this may sound great for someone else, but maybe you're thinking it's not for you. What if you can't or won't do it, or your partner can't or won't do it? It doesn't mean the relationship is over. Plenty of people have okay relationships and they accept this as "good enough" because they aren't willing to be that vulnerable or they don't want to be that intimate. Maybe they just aren't ready. Maybe they have some inner healing to do first.

Or, maybe you decide you want this kind of relationship, but not with the person you're with now. That's okay, too. Not every relationship is meant to last for a lifetime. Most probably aren't. For some of us, it takes a few tries to find the one we're willing to go to this level with.

Ending relationships is hard, but you can love someone and still not want to continue the relationship. Someone can love you and still not want to continue the relationship, and if you're on the receiving end of that, there's nothing you can do about it. You can only control how you respond. In the end, nothing is permanent, and we all have to say good-bye at some point. If you can continue to love and support someone after the relationship is over, then you will know you have mastered learning how not to blame someone else for something that was your responsibility. Some people just aren't designed to coexist over the long term.

All relationships have problems. They're made out of humans, after all. But they are far more successful and satisfying if you both approach them from an abundance perspective. Improving a relationship isn't about what you can get from a relationship. It's about what you can give to it. How can you add value to the relationship? Instead of asking *What can I get?* or *What's missing?* we asked ourselves *What can I do? What can I add?*

If you approach a relationship as an obligation, that's coming from a place of lack. Who wants a partnership that feels like a job? Nobody. When you approach partnerships, or any relationships, as a privilege and an honor, that's coming from a place of abundance. Your mindset is "I *get* to be in this relationship! I *get* to have interactions with this person. I *get* to know this person completely, body and soul, authentically in their truth. I *get* to be held by this person authentically in my truth." It's an absolute gift.

YOUR MIRRORS

An exercise that has really helped us reframe issues is to consider that everyone we have problems with is a mirror for our own self-exploration. This applies to any relationship—romantic partners, parents, children, friends, colleagues . . . everyone is a potential mirror for you. When someone makes you angry or irritable or triggers you, they are a mirror for what you are projecting onto them. We project onto the world, and especially onto the people we love, what is within us, so no matter the issue, it reflects back on you and it's up to you to take responsibility for it.

Even something as small as how your partner loads the dishwasher or puts on the toilet paper roll is about you if it generates a negative feeling. Explore it. Own it, feel it, and move on so you can get back to the business of creating the relationships you desire.

Whether you've known someone for five minutes or fifty years, they can be your mirror. Every time you look at someone else and think, *You aren't making me happy,* what you're really saying is, *I'm not making me happy.* When you think, *Why aren't you being romantic with me?* what you're really saying is, *Why aren't I being romantic with you?* When you think, *Why do you have to keep doing XYZ?* what you're really saying is, *What about XYZ bothers me so much?*

What an opportunity, to have such clear access to your inner being.

The Source of Happiness

You don't have to be in any relationship you don't want to be in. It's your choice, but relationships are an opportunity for self-development, and without them, you're not going to learn as much about yourself. There is always more personal work each of us can do to be better people, in and out of relationships. There is always a different way of seeing things, and there is always the opportunity to respond rather than react.

All relationships have stages. In romantic partnerships, there's that honeymoon period where everything's hot and sexy and you're just so happy, you can't take your hands off each other. Eventually that all shifts because life happens. We've been together for twenty-one years (so far!), and we've been married for eighteen of those years. A lot has happened during that time. The romance and passion can ebb and flow as the shit piles on and the mundanity of life takes over, but that initial feeling is under there somewhere, like an underground stream beneath the bedrock of the relationship, and you can always drill down and dip back into it if you choose.

That requires daily work, although we like to think of it as daily play—the teasing, the flirting, the fun, the physical touch, the appreciation. All of that bolsters a partnership and strengthens your bond, and it doesn't have to feel like work. It's a buffer against all the stress that can bring you down with work and family problems and bills and the dog that threw up all over the kitchen floor or whatever it is that comes at you every day. It can be a shelter.

Every day you can choose each other again. Every day you can take responsibility for yourself. Every day you can ask yourself what you can bring to the partnership. Every day you can show up as the person you want to be in that relationship. Every day you can be playful, loving, supportive, caring, giving. Every day you can touch each other, smile at each other, encourage each other, and forge a stronger bond that makes your relationship more resilient. Every day you can choose to be happy, not because the other person made you happy, but because you know how to find happiness within.

The last thing we want to say is that if you're in a relationship—any kind of relationship—and it's really not what you want, you don't need to turn around and go straight into another relationship. What you probably need is to work on your relationship with yourself. Get to know who you are. Get to know what you want. Get to know what makes you happy, gives you joy, and makes you feel alive. When you're open and receptive and out there being you, you will know who you are, and then you'll attract the person who's right for you.

The next level of human relationships beyond personal relationships is the tribal, and to us, that is the culmination, not just of health but of a meaningful life. That brings us to our final pillar.

PRIMAL UPRISING LITMUS TEST

> Are you completely honest in your relationships?
> Do you take full responsibility for your own happiness?
> Do you feel whole outside of your relationships?
> Do you feel free to be who you really are in your relationships?
> Can you be all aspects of your true self with your partner?
> Do you accept everything about who your partner is, without judgment?
> How is your relationship with yourself?

PART VIII
THE
TRIBAL
PILLAR

Call it a clan, call it a network, call it a tribe, call it a family. Whatever you call it, whoever you are, you need one.

—Jane Howard

17

FREE TO GATHER

> Two of the behaviors that set early humans apart were the systematic sharing of food and altruistic group defense . . . The earliest and most basic definition of community—of tribe—would be the group of people that you would both help feed and help defend. A society that doesn't offer its members the chance to act selflessly in these ways isn't a society in any tribal sense of the word; it's just a political entity that, lacking enemies, will probably fall apart on its own.
>
> —Sebastian Junger

We are all tribal people at heart—social animals who form groups meant to help support, feed, protect, and defend each other. We realize that many find the use of this word problematic, or even offensive, but we use the word very intentionally, with love and respect. The word *tribe* does not belong to any specific culture. The term originated in ancient Rome as *tribus,* which denoted a division within the state, and was later used in biblical texts to describe the divisions of the early Israelites. The word appears with this meaning in Middle English in the thirteenth century and has also been used historically to describe any group of people who live and work together in a shared geographical area with a common culture, dialect, and religion, and a strong sense of unity.

Tribes represented the stage of evolution between bands and nations, and as a movement that looks back in order to move forward, we use it as a word of connection, not division. In the Paleosphere, we are like-minded and share a common dialect and belief system. We are unified by those beliefs and dialects, which is why we consider ourselves a tribe in the best and most incredible sense of the world, and that is something innate in our humanness that goes back to our ancestors and roots . . . *everyone's* ancestors and roots. There have been tribes in every ancient culture, and when we speak of modern tribes, we refer to that sense of small-group unity. We have the utmost respect for the word *tribe* and would never use it in a demeaning or derogatory manner. We actually looked for another word to use and kept coming back to the word *tribe* to describe our Paleo f(x) family, but based on our research, we decided that was the most fitting and accurate word. That extends to its use in this book, so we hope you will read it with that spirit and intention in mind, because gathering in groups is still part of our psychology. For millions of years, that common interest was survival, which necessitated acting in the best interest of the tribe rather than selfishly. There's no denying that instinct still lives in us. We don't feel whole unless we feel like part of a group.

In his illuminating videos about tribalism, philosophy professor Kevin deLaplante describes how tribal psychology is built into us.[43] We aren't well designed for individual survival, but we are well designed to survive in a group, and what he calls our "groupishness" has been the key to our success as a species. We were able to hunt very large animals by hunting together, using cooperative strategies and division of labor. This helped our brains evolve, with tribe members specializing and getting better and more adept at certain tasks.

You can still see these traits today in any group of people with a common interest who have to work together, cooperating to utilize the best skills of each individual. Another trait of tribes is to act in the best interest of the group over the individual, and although we aren't often in the kinds of survival situations of our ancient ancestors, that impulse still lives within us, especially when survival is threatened.

One example of this is in the military, during wartime. Keith experienced this, especially after he didn't have it anymore. He says that being deployed is like a hellish version of the movie *Groundhog Day* . . . every day is the same, or some different variation of hell, and the only thing that keeps you going is the idea that you have your family to go back to. You don't think about the close interactions you have with your fellow soldiers until you get home, but then you do and you feel the loss of the tribe you never really recognized you were a part of.

He remembers coming back from deployment and feeling like he was in the lap of luxury at home, compared to where he had been, and yet, he was miserable. He couldn't understand why. Nobody was threatening to blow his head off, but at the same time, nobody was depending on him for their survival anymore, and he wasn't putting his own survival in the hands of anyone else. His tribe had dissolved. Keith remembers calling his best friend and saying, "Dude, I've been home for seventy-two hours and all I can think about is going back."

You can't replace that close connection with another human being who has your life in his hands. It's an adrenaline rush to be so close to death, and that triggers an emotional bond with the people who go through it with you. Keith says that time in the military was when he felt the most alive. Back then, he wasn't thinking about what the military action was about. There wasn't time for intellectualizing. He had to survive. Now, he can look back and see Big Military's agenda, but on the ground, it wasn't about the big picture. It was about the tribe, and it was intoxicating. He thinks this is one reason he went into entrepreneurship— it was the closest thing he could find to working on the high wire without a net.

Natural disaster situations are much the same. Look at communities experiencing a hurricane, flood, tornado, tsunami, or major earthquake, and you'll see the best of humanity emerging. People have frequently been known to take great risks to save others in their communities, including people they don't know, or at least to reach out and help the group to survive at the expense of individual resources.

Before Keith and Michelle were married, Keith lived on the coast of North Carolina, in a hurricane-prone area. In 1999, it experienced two category 5 hurricanes back to back: Hurricanes Denis and Floyd. The hurricane path just happened to follow a river near his house and the storm surge pushed water up over the banks of the river, then the hurricane stalled over the town and dumped a huge amount of additional water. It all converged and boom, they had a five-hundred-year flood.

Keith's small college town was totally cut off from the rest of the world, with no way to get in or out. All the airports were shut down. It was like Armageddon. The stores were empty and the water and electricity were shut off. There was no internet, no cable, and no other form of communication. The only radio station that was up and running and had enough oomph to reach the town was the one playing AM "oldies" from the 1950s. (Every time Keith hears a song from the '50s, he feels like he's back in that moment.)

But instead of suffering alone, all the neighborhoods came together— this person had a generator, that person had extra room in the generator-powered freezer, one family had meat to share, another had clean water. It was the only way they could all survive until the National Guard flew in to deliver water. When Keith looks back at that time, he considers it another memorable time in his life, in the best ways.

Even in the absence of a tight-knit group, there are always stories about the person who ran into a burning building to save someone, or jumped into icy waters to save someone, or braved some other hazardous condition for the sake of rescuing someone. We still have the instinct to save one another's lives, but since our lives are generally so safe, we don't have to use it much and it has faded into the background of consciousness. Yet, the instinct to form tribes remains in the forefront of human behavior.

Modern Tribes

Anything that connects people into a group can be a kind of tribe—people who root for the same team, people who worship the same religion together, people who share a passion or a hobby that has its own subculture, or people who have the same political beliefs all display qualities commonly considered to be tribal. If you get a positive feeling of belonging, understanding, and support, whether physical or emotional, from a group of people who share your beliefs or passions, that's your tribe. Those feel like your people.

Consider a sports team. They often behave like a military platoon at "war," and the bond between team members can be emotionally intense. You might not have anything in common with the other people on your team, but you all have the same goal. You are one unit, and societal constructs of division between people of different socioeconomic groups, race, creed, or whatever don't matter in the heat of the game. All that matters on the field is who's competent and who you can depend on to get the job done. It shares elements with a survival situation, and team members will often act altruistically for the good of the team. When a team member acts selfishly, it's considered bad sportsmanship at best.

There are countless other examples. People form groups so naturally that even when they are only loosely connected, people think of them as important. Families are a kind of tribe. Some neighborhoods form tribes. A band of musicians is a kind of tribe. So are people who work together, or people with the same profession (doctors, lawyers, writers, entrepreneurs). We've formed multiple micro-tribes in this way. One of our tribes is based on soulpreneurship. One is based on biohacking. One is our Burning Man family. One is our wealth dynamics family, and one is our Christian tribe. One works together with us in the plant medicine space to evolve and ascend and become better humans. Some of the people in each of these groups overlap, but there is a core group of about twenty people we consider our most intimate and essential soul family. These are the die-hard Keith and Michelle fans, and we are the die-hard fans of each of them.

But not everybody has what feels like a tribe. People can now go for days, weeks, months at a time without ever communicating face to face with another human being in any meaningful way. We can be lonely in the middle of a crowded city, and that is an unnatural and unhealthy state for humans. We think this is one reason for the rise in mental illnesses like depression and anxiety. We simply weren't designed for our survival needs to be met by technology rather than by other people.

This is one of the main problems we sought to repair when we started Paleo f(x), and it's the one comment we hear over and over about what people love the most about it—the opportunity to mingle in real life and in real time, for that feeling of support and like-mindedness about health. We say, "Come for the event. Stay for the tribe." We have witnessed firsthand what becoming part of a tribe can do for people. A few years ago, we got a letter written by a 17-year-old girl who had a lot of allergies and sensitivities. She was very limited in what she could eat and had been battling eating disorders all her life. When she goes out with her friends, she has to ask about every food she wants to eat. Sometimes, she said, it was easier for her to just sit there drinking water.

She wrote that she had been coming to the conference every year for the past five years because she finally felt like she had a place to go where she felt like part of a group. Like she belonged. At Paleo f(x), she said she felt that she had a home, a community, a tribe. She said she never felt normal anywhere else because of all the extreme things she has to do to stay healthy. When we read that, Michelle burst into tears. She said, "This is the whole reason we do this—so people can feel normal together."

This is what the like-minded, supportive group can do for an individual: Let them know they are normal. *You* are normal. It's the system that isn't normal. What's normal is to have respect for our bodies, for our health, for our food, for our environment, and for each other. When you find other people who also believe that, it's a great feeling.

Your tribe doesn't have to be Paleo f(x) (although you are always welcome to join us!). It can be any group that shares your values and makes you feel like you can be yourself, in your full expression of yourself. When this is how you feel, you will naturally act altruistically because the preservation of the tribe will be so important to you.

The Shadow Side of Tribe

We are meant to gather, but there is a shadow side to tribe, and the word *tribalism* has been co-opted to describe it. Technically, tribalism is just a word to describe the nature of being in a tribe, but when the bonds of a tribe result in extreme polarization, what was unifying can become dangerously divisive.

Whenever you add an "ism," you introduce a more divisive mindset, whether positive or negative: communism, rugged individualism, socialism, capitalism, humanism, fascism, populism, feminism—some of these terms may seem threatening to you and others may seem noble, but the "ism" within them contains an implicit "us versus them" mentality. It is polarizing.

Polarization isn't always bad. It's a matter of degree. All tribes, teams, groups, squads, or whatever you want to call them, have some polarization—that's kind of the point. The very nature of finding those with common beliefs implies that there are those who don't share those beliefs. There is tribe, and there is not-tribe, or not-our-tribe. This still isn't necessarily bad until those in a tribe begin to attach moral superiority to their beliefs, and moral inferiority or immorality or some other bad quality to those who don't share those beliefs. This can lead to shaming, ostracism, control, shunning, and violence.

The more we move away from the noble notion of tribe as a whole with light and dark in it, toward normalizing its shadow side as acceptable (like the many ways we excuse or overlook violence when perpetrated by someone in our own "tribe" while decrying it from those in a different "tribe"), the less opportunity we have to integrate and learn to control that shadow side. We all have negative thoughts and feelings, but nobody has to act on them. Instead, we can recognize them for what they are: symptoms of privilege, systemic sexism or racism, or simple ignorance. Seeing them for what they are can disempower them so they don't control our behavior. The shadow side of tribe isn't something to rationalize away or oversimplify. It's something to acknowledge and manage. In our modern world, differences are most likely to be of opinions (convictions), and letting those differences be divisive sacrifices the many benefits of unity in the broader sense.

THE ORIGIN OF MORALITY

One theory about the origin of morality is that morality is based on what advances social interactions, constructs, and behaviors, or what helps humans work together, cooperate, and help and protect each other.[44] This is one explanation for why we have decided, culturally, that killing, coveting, stealing, anger, violence, and so on. (the list of "sins" in any culture or religion) are "bad": They are immoral because they hurt group solidarity and function. They weaken the social construct by causing internal division, or by putting members of the group at risk of injury or death through the violence that can result from extreme polarization.

Prosocial behaviors, like love, cooperation, sharing, and sacrifice, are considered "good" because they help group members understand each other better, exercise compassion, and develop more skills to increase resources, health, and reproduction. They benefit the tribe. We think this is a great lens through which to determine "goodness" or "badness." Is it unifying or divisive? Does it increase health or decrease it? Does it support or undermine? Does it build or does it destroy?

Forming groups based on our differences can cause us to forget how much we are all the same.

What we propose is the creation of discerning and intelligent groups that are internally strong, connected, and supportive, but who are also capable of understanding that differences aren't bad and that those in other groups who have different views are still fellow humans. Any two groups of people *always* have more in common than they have differences, if you step back and look at the broad perspective. It's just a matter of where you put your focus. We are all members of the human tribe, and all our internal divisions are just subgroups that help us connect with like-minded people.

The ideal of gathering is to encourage survival and the pursuit of human potential, not to fight and destroy each other.

Reinstating Rituals and Rites of Passage

Another aspect of tribal culture that we have largely lost is the importance of rituals and rites of passage to mark the passing of time and life stages. The rituals we have today are shells of their former selves. What were once sacred rituals have become for-profit holidays. Rites of passage like bar mitzvahs and sweet sixteens have largely become parties with no real meaning. This has contributed, we believe, to generations of people who never really grew up or understood what it means to be an adult, and millions of adults who no longer feel the sacred nature of life or the passage of time.

In many different native cultures, children (typically boys) were given some kind of challenge, journey, or quest to complete in order to transition into adulthood. The challenges were often dangerous, but that was the point. When (if) they returned, they re-joined the group as adults. But try that today with your eleven-year-old son and you'll get child protective services knocking on your door. Instead, we throw parties, give presents, eat food. We've made adolescence safer (arguably), but less meaningful. The stakes are much lower so it feels less important to become an adult. In fact, why bother?

We remember when fifteen-year-old Laura Dekker sailed around the world alone, to follow the trip her parents had taken twenty years before. Leading up to that successful voyage was a series of court cases in which authorities kept intervening to stop her. Once, on a practice voyage to England from her home in the Netherlands, the authorities put her in foster care until her father came to pick her up. She and her father both knew she was capable of the journey, and they both knew the risks, but the local government decided they knew better than to let her engage in this fantastic rite of passage. (Fortunately, she was finally able to do it. Her journey lasted over five hundred days and is captured in a 2013 documentary called *Maidentrip*.)

We also remember the uproar when a woman in Washington, DC, allowed her nine-year-old son to take a thirty-minute train trip by himself, a trip he had taken many times before with an adult. The conductor stopped the train and refused to move it until the police arrived.

We've heard countless stories of social services called on parents who let their children try to do things alone, like play in the park unaccompanied, go to the store, or walk home from school. It's not a simple issue—it's a dangerous world, and many children are neglected, victimized, and abused. There are agencies to watch out for that and to protect children. At the same time, many perfectly capable and mature children aren't allowed to do things they should be able to try on their own, if they feel ready and their parents are involved and supportive. Many of the rites of passage ancient cultures practiced played a valuable role in creating a boundary between childhood and adulthood, shifting more responsibilities onto children as they grew older. Today, children aren't often given much responsibility until they're thrown into the adult world, and that's a harsh transition—much worse, in our opinion, than a rite of passage that builds a child's confidence so they feel ready to enter adulthood.

As Canadian psychologist Jordan Peterson says, "Too much protection devastates the developing soul." Young people clamor for responsibility. They crave it—even if they complain! It makes them feel accomplished. They want to prove, to others and to themselves, that they are transitioning into adults. We should be able to give this to our young adults. It's a move toward building a better world in the future, run by more capable people.

Keith remembers when he used to have to do manual labor jobs in the summer when he was 14 and 15 years old. He remembers how empowering it felt to get up in the morning and slug back a cup of coffee with his uncles, then join the men going out to the jobsite. He felt like a real adult during those summers of hard work, more than he did in school (although football was its own sort of ritual for growth). That's not so young, historically. Centuries ago, people (or at least men) were considered capable adults at fifteen. In many ancient cultures, fifteen-year-olds were joining the hunt, helping with the gathering and food preparation, and taking care of (or already having their own) children. We prolong that now, and although there are benefits to slowing down the clock and letting kids be kids longer, we still have that need for marking that shift from childhood to adulthood. Adolescence is confusing enough, and rituals and rites of passage can help give structure and make sense of that confusion.

Somewhere there is a line between constantly living in fear that something bad might happen to your child and taking risks that create periodic opportunities for growth and maturity. Every time we drive a child in a car or take a child on an airplane, it's a risk, but it's a risk we don't usually think about. If anybody really stopped to think about the odds of getting into a car accident and becoming completely debilitated or dying, nobody would ever go anywhere.

We believe in putting these risks in perspective and teaching children how to take on responsibility for themselves and their own lives. Just because we don't have the same rituals and rites of passage we once had doesn't mean we can't create new ones that help us grow and experience life in a more meaningful way. In the next chapter, we'll look at some ways to do that, along with ways to build your own tribe or soul family.

PRIMAL UPRISING LITMUS TEST

> Do you have people in your life who make you feel comfortable enough to be yourself?
> Do you have people in your life who share your passions?
> What rituals do you practice already?
> Did you experience any rites of passage in adolescence?

18

BUILDING TRIBAL RESILIENCE

It is the nature of the mind that makes individuals kin.

—Isaac Asimov

W e can't imagine life without our tribe, or what we call our family of choice, life team, or soul family. These are the people we can call at 3:00 a.m. and no matter what's going on, they'll get out of bed and come to help us. We would do (and have done) the same for any of them. Nobody in our soul family will ever be homeless or hungry, and none of us will ever have abundance while others in our tribe have lack. These are the people we "do life" with—our "ride or die" soul family. We play together, grow together, and work together to serve the common good. They serve us and we serve them. We have each other's backs, and we have each other's best interest in mind.

Our tribe isn't so much held together because we all have exactly the same beliefs. We don't. It's a bond based on spiritual kinship. When we are with these people, we feel our own unlimited potential because they see our limitlessness and we see their limitlessness. We push each other upward and upward, evolving and transcending ourselves constantly. It took some time to build our soul family, but it has made our lives more complete.

So how do you find and build a soul family that can do these things for you? How do you find like-minded people that you can form strong bonds with, so much so that you are willing to do anything for them and they are willing to do anything for you? Let's explore some options.

Creating Your Soul Family

To begin creating a family of choice begins with understanding what you are passionate about. What makes you feel alive? What matters to you? What reflects your values? We have a friend in Salt Lake City who is part of a "doomsday group." The group is a band of twenty or so people, each with a highly honed set of specific skills (our friend's is navigation, rock climbing, and general survival skills) designed with overlap redundancy so that the band as a whole would be able to survive just about any situation. When it all goes down, when survival suddenly seems dire, they know where to meet. It might sound morbid, but their bond is strong because they are all dedicated to a common passion (and just think of the fantastic collection of survival skills these people now have at their disposal!).

When you express who you are and do what you want to be doing, you'll naturally attract others who feel the same about whatever it is you consider to be important in your life. Form or join supportive groups based on what interests you.

Another way to begin is to take stock of the people who are currently in your life. Do they fall into groups? Do you have work friends, friends from the past, friends who share a similar interest? Which ones feel the most natural for you? Where can you really be yourself? Where do you feel the most accepted? Which groups are the most fun, interesting, stimulating, or comfortable to be with? This can be the beginning of a tribe that can grow.

If you struggle to think of people in your life who fit this description, it may be time to expand your circles. Go online to find people with similar interests. Join some groups. Reach out. You could also take a class, join a club, go to religious services, go to community events. When you step outside of yourself, you will be more likely to put out the energy that will attract like-minded people. Keep looking. Don't give up. This is a matter of health.

Once you have a group (or a few groups) in mind, you can cultivate them. Envision how you might want to interact with these people. Suggest getting together to do something you all enjoy. Assess how it goes. Maybe you all like to travel and you can plan trips together. Maybe you love to have complex discussions, or you all like to cook and have dinner parties, or go to concerts, or hike, or dance, or meditate together. Whatever it is, test the waters of gathering.

The more time you spend together, the more a soul family will organically form. Prioritize these gatherings. Don't let life get in the way of something that is food for your soul. Talk. Share. Do. Get to know each other better. Learn what each other's goals and dreams are. Ask each other questions. If money was no object, what would you all be doing? Sharing feelings builds intimacy and connection. You may find that some people fall away from the core group, while others may appear who fit right in.

As your soul family grows closer, ask yourself whether you have the impulse to give to the tribe, or whether you have more of an attitude that you should get something from it. If you were in a survival situation, would those people help you? If they were, would you want to help them? How can you show up and be of value to the group? The more you do this, the more others in the group are likely to follow your example. Maybe others are already there, and you can be inspired by them.

Evolving Your Soul Family

Soul families change over time and so do you. That means yours may have an expiration date just as another one is rising up to meet you. Sometimes a group becomes too polarized or too one-pointed and it can lose resilience. Sometimes a group becomes too diffuse to have a connection anymore. To cultivate your tribal resilience, stay attuned to the health of your group and be open to letting it evolve naturally, even if that means it disperses.

To keep a tribe growing requires an influx of new people and new ideas. Otherwise, any group of like-minded people can become an echo chamber. Sharing common beliefs can be a form of stress relief, especially in a divisive world, and that's great, but at a certain point it can begin to reinforce singular opinions without room for different ways of seeing.

Keith in particular feels uncomfortable in these echo chamber situations. He's seen it happen at strength and conditioning conferences, for example—people get tunnel vision about one ideology or point of view, and Keith feels that it sucks the life out of whatever it is they think is the "only way." In a few years, whatever business or movement the idea was about is usually dead because they never brought in any alternative points of view. They didn't evolve.

We were determined not to let this happen at Paleo f(x), which is why we are always seeking to bring in people with alternative points of view, just to rattle the cage a bit. For example, we have people with a lot of different ideas about what constitutes a paleo diet, and we've even brought in vegans to keep everybody on their toes, ideologically. This doesn't threaten the tribe. It makes it stronger and more adaptable because it gets us all to question our beliefs and argue our points, and sometimes we even change our minds.

BRANDON YAGER SAYS . . .

Brandon Yager, along with his wife Deb, is our neurolinguistic programming trainer, and he has a story about crabs in a bucket, as an analogy for determining who should be in your tribe. It's a way to think about who is lifting you up and who is holding you down. Here's how he tells it:

> Right after high school, I worked up in Alaska as a fishing guide boat boy. I cleaned fish. I cleaned boats. It was a beautiful job for me to learn about all the ways the world works, especially the fishing life in remote Alaska, which I still believe is truly the last frontier.

I worked up there with a guy named Art. Art was a great teacher and taught me everything I needed to know about catching halibut and king salmon and netting shrimp and prawn and how to set crab pots. We'd fish and net all day, then ready the crab pots and throw them overboard. We'd come back later in the day or sometimes the next morning and bring in the haul.

At 18 I was pretty naive and didn't have anything much about life figured out. I certainly didn't know about crabs. The first time I hauled out a crab pot, it had only one male crab in it. We threw the females back out to sea and threw the single male in a large retaining bucket on deck. No sooner had I tossed him in the bucket than that little guy just crawled right up out of that bucket and onto the floor of the boat. I was like, Whoa, what's going on here? Things move fast on a boat deck, so I grabbed the runaway crab and tossed him back in the bucket as another pot was hauled on board. This one was full of all kinds of crabs, probably six or seven of them in there. All of them males. We threw all of them in the bucket with the runaway crab. I looked all over for a lid; something to keep all the crabs from a jailbreak. Art laughed. "We don't need a lid, son," he said. "Watch." And wouldn't you know it, one of those crabs was almost on its way out of the bucket. And another crab reached up and pulled him right back in. And I was like, Huh. Look at that.

So this "crabs in a bucket" thing isn't just a made-up story. It's real. I've seen it for myself. Crabs won't let other crabs flee their captive environment. It's not malicious; they just don't know any other way to be. And people can be the same way.

So who are your crabs? Who is holding you back? And what bucket are they keeping you in, when you know you have to climb out to be free? Those "crabs" are the people you might want to winnow from your tribe.

Making Rituals Sacred Again

What if you could make the rituals you already have in your life feel more meaningful and sacred? One way we do that is by celebrating milestones and the passage of time with our soul families. One of our favorite annual rituals is Orphan Thanksgiving. We invite our soul family and people in our community who don't have family close by. Our friends invite others who might be alone, and we invite our own family members, too. This has become a treasured event for our community, and it grows each year. Here are some other ideas for reinstating more rituals into your life, and making them more sacred and meaningful:

- Turn a holiday into a service day. Volunteer at a food kitchen, deliver food to families in need, help build a Habitat for Humanity house (or build it ahead of time and gift it on the holiday), or look into other service opportunities in your city or town. Serving others brings sacred energy to what could otherwise feel selfish and indulgent.

- When you celebrate, put the emphasis on people and experiences rather than things and money. Celebrate individuality by asking each person to bring something to the ritual that reflects who they are. Accept it without judgment.

- Make traditional foods for traditional celebrations, or begin a tradition of having the same foods at each celebration. Food rituals can trigger memories and make the celebration feel more emotionally significant over time. Look back to your own cultural heritage for traditional recipes and foods.

- Families are a sort of tribe. Start a family reunion tradition if you don't already have one. Make it a celebration of family traditions rather than an ego fest. Share photos, memories, and family lore, including stories about those from past generations, to generate a sense of the family's history. Or, make it a soul family reunion by inviting your nearest and dearest to gather every year. These can be an anchor for the year and something you look forward to for months.

- Create rites of passage for your own children. They can be more symbolic or involve an actual (reasonably safe) task, like camping out alone in the backyard or going on a special trip somewhere with a parent to do some kind of challenging activity (hiking, climbing a mountain, attending a learning conference, exploring a new city) as an experience to initiate them into adulthood. After they "pass" the ritual, ceremoniously grant them a few new adult privileges and responsibilities.

- When you have a life transition (marriage, childbirth, moving into a new home, kids moving out, even divorce), create a rite of passage around it to mark and remember the event. Even if it's a party, there can be a serious and solemn aspect to mark the transition. Light a candle, say a prayer, bless the new child or place, or do something to symbolize the joining or un-joining.

- Create a ritual around the turning of the seasons or the solstices and equinoxes. There are many ancient seasonal rituals you could explore. Look back to what your own ancestors might have done and see if you can create some kind of modern facsimile.

- Make New Year's Eve about more than champagne and revelry. This can be a sacred rite of passage into the next year, marked by honoring the past and setting intentions for the present. Write down your intentions, then throw them in a fire or put them in a special place where you can return to them throughout the year as a reminder.

Most important is to personalize your rituals and rites of passage so they feel meaningful to you. We can't overstate how much value this brings to life.

Now that we have come to the end of the seven pillars, let's turn to organizational and inspirational concerns. In the last section of this book, we'll help you figure out how to integrate the seven pillars into your life, and we hope to send you off with a bit of paleo fervor, as we give you a snapshot of what our world could look like beyond the zoo.

PRIMAL UPRISING LITMUS TEST

> Who is in your soul family? Do you have more than one tribe?
> How might you curate your tribe to strengthen it?
> How can you serve the group?
> How can others in your group complement your strengths, interests, or skills?
> If someone in your group was in danger, would you come to their rescue, even if it meant risking your own safety? Would they come to your rescue?
> What are ways you can create more rituals in your life?
> What are rites of passage that could be meaningful to you and your family?

Of course, we are both all about the amazing, delicious, fantastic paleo food that helps us feel stronger and sharper every day. Beyond that, Keith prioritizes exercise, while Michelle's approach is more emotional and spiritual, focusing on stress management and meditation. Start with food and expand from there—you can think of the pillars as areas to tackle in order, or you can jump around as if they are spokes on a wheel, but the essentials are easy. Here's a recap of what we've suggested throughout this book so far:

- Eat real, whole food: vegetables, animal protein, roots/tubers, nuts/seeds, natural fats, and fruit.
- Move as much as you can: walk, sprint, swim, lift, carry, push, pull, drag, flow, do sports.
- Sleep seven to nine hours a night.
- Manage your stress with meditation.
- Think for yourself and notice when outside forces are attempting to manipulate your opinions and attention.
- Be discerning.
- Accept your emotions and feel your feelings.
- Believe in something bigger than yourself.
- Treat money like energy and let it flow into your life.
- Love others as much as you can.
- Be with people. Look them in the eye. Listen.
- Touch, hold hands, make love, and hug your loved ones every day.
- Let other people be your mirror.
- Value, be there for, and depend on your tribe.
- Know that we are all one, and that although we have our differences, what's more important is what we all have in common.
- Seek freedom.

See how simple it is? See how beautiful your life could be, if you live by the pillars and prioritize what really matters in life? Simple doesn't mean easy, and that's why it helps to keep your goals in mind. You are training for a stronger, better, more resilient future. You are training for your own longevity, cognition, resilience, and good mood. And you are training to be part of something bigger.

PART IX
PLAYBOOK FOR THE UPRISING

The only way to deal with an unfree world is to become so absolutely free that your very existence is an act of rebellion.

—Albert Camus

19

BASIC TRAINING

In preparing for battle, I have always found that plans are use-
less, but planning is indispensable.

—Dwight D. Eisenhower

The purpose of the seven pillars is to get you ready for your primal
uprising, whether that uprising remains within the boundaries of your
personal life, or extends to your family or community, or to activism
on a broader scale. We want you to be the best that you can be, in every
aspect, and in this chapter we want to help you start doing it for real.

To inspire you, we tell you how each of us organizes our own lives to
achieve our health and freedom goals: what we do, how we plan, and how
we stay focused. At the end of the chapter, we give you some templates to
help you start organizing the aspects from this book that you choose to
integrate into your own life, whether you are going for a total overhaul or
you want to start slow, changing just a few things at a time and waiting to
see how well they work. Your life, your style, your pace—as you'll see, we
each "do life" a bit differently, and there are as many ways to pursue the
seven pillars as there are people. We hope this chapter will help you figure
out the best way for you to do *you*. Remember, paleo is flexible! What matters is that you are moving forward and that your plan is enjoyable so you
want to keep doing it.

PART IX
PLAYBOOK
FOR THE
UPRISING

The only way to deal with an unfree world is to become so absolutely free that your very existence is an act of rebellion.

—Albert Camus

19

BASIC TRAINING

In preparing for battle, I have always found that plans are use-
less, but planning is indispensable.

—Dwight D. Eisenhower

The purpose of the seven pillars is to get you ready for your primal
uprising, whether that uprising remains within the boundaries of your
personal life, or extends to your family or community, or to activism
on a broader scale. We want you to be the best that you can be, in every
aspect, and in this chapter we want to help you start doing it for real.

To inspire you, we tell you how each of us organizes our own lives to
achieve our health and freedom goals: what we do, how we plan, and how
we stay focused. At the end of the chapter, we give you some templates to
help you start organizing the aspects from this book that you choose to
integrate into your own life, whether you are going for a total overhaul or
you want to start slow, changing just a few things at a time and waiting to
see how well they work. Your life, your style, your pace—as you'll see, we
each "do life" a bit differently, and there are as many ways to pursue the
seven pillars as there are people. We hope this chapter will help you figure
out the best way for you to do *you*. Remember, paleo is flexible! What matters is that you are moving forward and that your plan is enjoyable so you
want to keep doing it.

Of course, we are both all about the amazing, delicious, fantastic paleo food that helps us feel stronger and sharper every day. Beyond that, Keith prioritizes exercise, while Michelle's approach is more emotional and spiritual, focusing on stress management and meditation. Start with food and expand from there—you can think of the pillars as areas to tackle in order, or you can jump around as if they are spokes on a wheel, but the essentials are easy. Here's a recap of what we've suggested throughout this book so far:

- Eat real, whole food: vegetables, animal protein, roots/tubers, nuts/seeds, natural fats, and fruit.
- Move as much as you can: walk, sprint, swim, lift, carry, push, pull, drag, flow, do sports.
- Sleep seven to nine hours a night.
- Manage your stress with meditation.
- Think for yourself and notice when outside forces are attempting to manipulate your opinions and attention.
- Be discerning.
- Accept your emotions and feel your feelings.
- Believe in something bigger than yourself.
- Treat money like energy and let it flow into your life.
- Love others as much as you can.
- Be with people. Look them in the eye. Listen.
- Touch, hold hands, make love, and hug your loved ones every day.
- Let other people be your mirror.
- Value, be there for, and depend on your tribe.
- Know that we are all one, and that although we have our differences, what's more important is what we all have in common.
- Seek freedom.

See how simple it is? See how beautiful your life could be, if you live by the pillars and prioritize what really matters in life? Simple doesn't mean easy, and that's why it helps to keep your goals in mind. You are training for a stronger, better, more resilient future. You are training for your own longevity, cognition, resilience, and good mood. And you are training to be part of something bigger.

PRIMAL WISDOM

Simplicity is the key to brilliance.
—BRUCE LEE

Let's start by setting some goals. Answer these questions, either right here in this book or in your journal:

1. The first, most urgent change I want to make to my physical health is:

2. The first thing I want to do to improve my mental health is:

3. Here's what I want to do to increase my emotional intelligence:

4. My plan for expanding and strengthening my spiritual life is to:

5. My most critical financial health goal right now is:

6. I'm ready to improve my relationships. This is the relationship I'm going to focus on first:

7. I want a tribe that I can rely on, and that can rely on me. Here are the people I think could be a part of my tribe. I'm going to focus on these people and be open to receiving them in my life:

8. This is how I would like my life to look one year from now (be as detailed as you can):

9. This will be me in five years:

10. This is me in ten years:

Now you have a basic game plan. To help you begin implementing and manifesting, we'll tell you some of what we do. We've written his book speaking together as one voice, but in the next two sections, we'll each "take the microphone" and tell you in our own words about how we organize our days, weeks, months, and years. (Note that we mention various products and services in our sections, not because we are telling you to buy or use them, but just because people always ask us what we use.)

Michelle's Schedule

I like to keep my schedule a little bit loose, rather than getting hung up on doing things exactly the same every day. Rigid schedules aren't possible with my lifestyle and aren't compatible with my personality.

No-Alarm Mornings

Back when I had a "regular job," before I became an entrepreneur, I used to wake up with an alarm, hit the snooze button, and end up being late. This created stress before I was even out of bed, which dumped a load of cortisol into my bloodstream. Next I would dive immediately into my email, which hijacked my brain, as I allowed other people's emergencies to become my emergencies. Within a few hours, as the cortisol worked its way out of my system, I'd have a huge crash and feel exhausted. I was never really able to regain control of my day.

Once I stopped doing that and took back my mornings for myself, I began to heal and was able to manage my stress much better. I'm almost never rushed in the morning so I never get that cortisol dump. Instead, I rev up gradually and get a nice, even cortisol rise, giving me energy to work and think when I need it most. Because of the difference it's made in my life, I strongly believe in bookending the days by putting mentally fortifying things into my brain instead of negative, stressful things.

Here's what I do now. Unless I have to catch a flight or have a meeting, I try never to wake up to an alarm clock. Alarms feel jarring to me, and that's not how I want to start my day. I might wake up naturally anywhere from 7:00 to 9:00 a.m., depending on how late I stayed up and what time of year it is (what time the sun rises). Sleep is so important for how the rest of my day goes that I prioritize it whenever I can.

I usually don't schedule myself for anything before 10:00 a.m., so I have that time from around 7:00 to 10:00 a.m. for myself. I try never to be rushed, so I can ease into the day on my own timeline to do what I feel like I need to do. The rest of my morning might look like this:

7:30 a.m.: Wake up, hydrate, then get a cup of coffee. I like a splash of A2 milk creamer (see page 62). I also take my thyroid medication.

7:45 a.m.: I take my coffee back to the bedroom, do my affirmations, then meditate for twenty to thirty minutes. I like to do guided meditations or visualizations, or sometimes I listen to a calming Spotify playlist. On the mornings that I don't feel like meditating, I'll read something uplifting or positive, or write in my journal if I'm inspired by something or want to work through something I've been thinking about. Some days, I'll use my friend Hal Elrod's Miracle Morning Savers.

HAL ELROD SAYS . . .

Hal Elrod is the bestselling author of *The Miracle Morning* and shares his wise words about the power of habit creation for changing your life and how habit stacking (attaching new habits to already established habits, like "After I brush my teeth every morning, I will drink a full glass of water") can help you change your life for the better:

> Habit stacking is arguably the single most important technique to master in order to create and sustain positive changes in your life. And the simpler the better. Simplicity means ease of repeatability, and repeatability is the key to compounding positive changes over time.

8:15 a.m.: I relax and take my time getting ready, doing my personal hygiene routine and getting dressed. That usually takes about twenty-five minutes.

8:45 a.m.: I take my morning supplements (my customized IDLifeWellness morning pack, of course!) and I track what supplements I took and how I slept the night before in my Daylio app (see the box on tracking).

9:00 a.m.: I take about an hour to relax and putter around. I might step outside for a few minutes to get sun on my face and help my brain wake up. Then I get my work set up and transition into work mode.

10:00 a.m.: I start working, fresh, positive, and ready for the day.

Breaking the Fast

I don't usually have breakfast. I practice intermittent fasting (page 89–90) on most days, so other than my coffee with a bit of cream (which isn't a hard-core way to fast, I realize!), I don't eat anything until about 1:00 or 2:00 p.m. At that time, I usually have some kind of protein- and fat-rich snack with fiber, like cashew butter on apple slices, a hard-boiled egg, or half an avocado. If I'm not actually hungry yet, I'll wait until I am. Sometimes that's not until dinnertime.

If you prefer to have breakfast, choose wisely. This is the fuel you'll be running on all day long. Generally, it's better to have protein and fat rather than carbohydrates. Morning carbs can trigger an insulin response and a blood sugar crash, making you tired and foggy. A protein-and-fat breakfast will keep your blood sugar steady so you'll have more energy. A small amount of fiber-rich carbs are best for evening because they can help you sleep better, which is why we usually reserve foods like potatoes as part of our dinner.

Calm Evenings

After work, we usually eat dinner around 5:30 or 6:00 p.m. I take digestive enzymes at every meal (because I have no gallbladder). Dinner is almost always gluten- and dairy-free, consisting of some grass-fed meat or wild-caught fish with a big salad, some cooked non-starchy vegetables, and some root vegetables. Very rarely I might have a glass of wine. I try to be finished eating by 6:30 or 7:00. If I'm finished eating by 7:00 p.m. and I don't eat again until 1:00 p.m. the next day, I've fasted for eighteen hours. This is the amount of time that makes me feel the best and the most energized.

After dinner, Keith and I usually spend time together watching documentaries, reading, or just talking and being together. It's our touch-base time. I've felt much happier and healthier since I stopped watching regular television and news about fifteen years ago. I don't go into a place of fear as often anymore. It doesn't mean I don't follow the news—we all get bombarded with it online and in social media. I don't like to get to the point where I don't know what's going on, but I dip my toe in carefully and I'm mindful of what my mind is consuming. When I do follow news online, I look for the most neutral sources I can, and I read everything with a healthy skepticism.

Every once in a while, if I'm still hungry, I'll have an evening snack. My favorite is heirloom popcorn made with avocado oil, with Himalayan salt and just a touch of grass-fed butter. Or I might have a couple of squares of very dark chocolate with 85 to 90 percent cacao. I am absolutely done eating by 8:00 p.m.

Before bed, I take my evening pack of vitamins and hormone-balancing and sleep-enhancing supplements, which has really helped me with hot flashes and being able to sleep through the night without night sweats.

Just before sleep, I do my affirmations again and then read something fun but not stimulating (like a novel). It has to be positive.

TRACKING

Every day, I track what I eat, what supplements I take, my alcohol consumption if any, my stress, how Keith and I are getting along, and anything different that happens, like hanging out with friends, traveling, having a beach day, taking a sauna and a cold shower, and so on. When I don't feel right, I can look back and figure out why. My favorite way to do this is with an app called Daylio, which is an online journal. I like it because it has customizable checkboxes I can check so I don't have to write down anything, plus room for notes if I want to mention anything unusual. I also track my sleep quality using the Oura ring and my movement with my Garmin watch. I don't rely on my tech trackers, though. What really matters is how I feel. My Oura ring might tell me I had a bad night's sleep, but if I feel great, I don't worry about it. I am the ultimate authority on me, not my tech.

Keith's Schedule

I try to find the middle way between blowing with the wind and having ironclad control—a little organization, a little flexibility—and tend to err on the side of ironclad, inspired by retired naval officer Jocko Willink, who says, "Discipline is freedom." Discipline doesn't have to mean obsessive restriction. It can simply mean unwavering focus. When you are disciplined to a task, you can achieve mastery. That mastery is freedom. If you are disciplined with your health and master the task of being healthy, then you will be more free and, as a result, healthy and harder to control.

No-Alarm Morning

Like Michelle, I usually get up without an alarm, around 7:00 to 7:30 a.m., but I don't force myself to get up before 7:30 unless there's something I have to do.

Right out of the gate, I drink twelve ounces of pure filtered water with a quarter teaspoon of Himalayan salt dissolved in it, to rehydrate and remineralize. I do this because I spend a lot of time outdoors in Austin, and that means I sweat a lot and lose a lot of minerals. People also sweat when they sleep (gross as that may sound). Your skin is always breathing, just as you are. That's why people so often wake up thirsty.

Next, I make a cup of strong black coffee—no cream, no butter, no oil, certainly no sugar—which gives me a cognitive boost. I like high-quality organic free-trade coffee. Coffee is my fuel and I drink it all day long, not just for sharper thinking but for the taste and the ritual.

I let the dogs out to do their thing and then I take my coffee upstairs to the office where my computer is. I always keep a document open on my computer that I use for free-flow writing (it's currently over seven hundred pages), and I begin.

Sacred Creativity Time

During this sacred morning creativity time, I write whatever comes to mind for about two hours. I don't email or text, just stay purely focused on creative output. That could be journaling, a blog post, or copy for an email I have to send. It could be ideating or writing fiction. I try not to have an agenda. This is one of those parts of my day when I stay flexible and go with the flow. About every twenty to thirty minutes, I go downstairs to refill my coffee, so I'm not sitting for the whole 2 hours.

I go until I run out of steam. If I hit a blank and sit there for a while twiddling my thumbs, I'll wait to see if something bubbles up. If it doesn't, I won't push it just to make it to two hours, but for me this time is non-negotiable and sets the tone for my day. Even if I miss something on the business side or have to reschedule, ultimately I know it will benefit me much more to have that creative time.

All Work and No Flow Makes Keith a Dull Boy

After that, I'll slide into doing regular business. First I go into my email and Slack (a communication app we use for work) and see if there is anything critical. I handle urgent things first and leave the least urgent for later in the afternoon. It's mind-energy management.

Next, I dive into social media with two purposes:

1. To get a quick feel for what's going on in the world. I have a news-feed set up in Twitter.

2. To look at what's going on from all different perspectives and all sides of the political spectrum so I don't get sucked into my own biases. I use social media to exercise my mental pillar and stay nimble. If something comes up that I need more time to think about, I'll put a note about it in my free-flow writing document, to work on the next morning.

On social media, our diverse group of friends constantly shares information with us. It could be anything about health and wellness to the wackiest conspiracy theories. It's all over the map and I love it! I also use it to track trends and guess what's going to be *big*. I saw keto coming—the concept had been around for decades, but I watched it begin to gain in popularity and now I'm watching it fall out of favor a bit. The one thing I didn't see coming was CrossFit. Back in 1997, I remember thinking, *Yeah, that's cool, but there's no way in hell the mainstream's ever going to go for it.* Little did I know! Of course, now that trend is fading, too. Tracking trends helps me ideate for Paleo f(x), and sometimes I help find our next great speaker that way.

This is all loosely organized so I can do any interviews or meetings during this time as needed. If I start to feel low on energy or craving something sweet, I'll have the IDLifeWellness Slim drink, which helps energize me and keeps me from wanting to snack on something I would regret. By noon or 1-ish, I'm getting to the point where I need a break, so I might work out and then have something to eat, like eggs and avocados (I usually fast until after my workout).

Priority Two: Working Out

My workout varies: Some days are very intense; others are easier. Some are long; some are short. I go by what feels right in the moment, but a typical workout might start with a long bike ride that acts as my warm-up as well as my meditation.

After my ride, I focus on strength training. Sometimes it's bodyweight-centric with basics like push-ups and pull-ups, and sometimes it looks like gymnastics. On other days I lift actual weights. I have a homemade kettlebell I made with threaded pipe forming a T-bar. I can put weights on it, making it as heavy as I want, and I can use this to do deadlifts or swings.

In rotating fashion (and over the course of two or three workouts), I cover all the basic categories of human movement: swinging, pushing, pulling, hinging, and driving. The varieties of push-ups, dips, pull-ups, rows, squats, and hinges are endless and for me, so creating and executing a new exercise combo is kinesthetic creativity. I mean, there are at least sixty different types of squats alone! Every day I try to do something different than I did the day before. It's important to cycle through your exercises because once the body adapts to a certain exercise, if that's all you do, you stop improving. I like to keep shaking it up. Sometimes that's as minor as trying a new hand position, changing speed, or altering the angle of execution.

Winding Down

After working out, I usually eat something. My eating, like my training, is difficult to classify; if I were pressed to describe it, I'd say it's "Mediterranean keto," low in carbs, high in healthy fats and protein. I compress my eating window from about 3:00 p.m. to about 9:00 p.m.—and during that time I've been known to eat pretty heartily! I usually clean my plate, and whatever Michelle doesn't finish. And then some. I want to be able to eat as much as I want, and this eating pattern works with my schedule. The eighteen-hour fast gives my body time to process everything.

At the end of the workday, I devote time to what I call those "brain-dead activities": no-effort tasks like answering mundane emails and dealing with regular business. I don't have any creativity left, so I do what doesn't require it. Then we have dinner.

After dinner, it's generally some kind of media consumption like watching documentaries with Michelle or reading a book, or we might have an entrepreneurial meetup at somebody's house. Sometimes we have dinner with friends. Most evenings, we'll take the dogs for a long walk.

I don't take much in the way of supplements beyond my customized IDLifeWellness pack (I know we keep mentioning it, but it is what we really do use). I usually take my morning pack with my first meal (so it's really more like an afternoon pack) and my evening pack after dinner.

Basically, my schedule can be jam-packed and rigid or free-flowing and all over the map, and I'm totally cool with it either way. My two big nonnegotiables are those two hours of creativity in the morning and some form of daily exercise, because of how much value they add to my life.

Weekly, Monthly, Yearly

Back to our unified voice because our weekly, monthly, and yearly schedules are pretty similar since we work and live together. Mondays are different for us than the rest of the week. That's when we have back-to-back meetings with our team from 10:00 a.m. to around 5:00 p.m. After work, we usually try to have dinner with friends. On the weekends, our schedule can vary because we often go on a retreat or travel.

CLEARING THE LIST

At the end of every week, usually on Sunday evening, Michelle looks back over the past week and consults her journal for notes about all the things she wanted to do, people she wanted to talk to, things she wanted to research, documentaries she wanted to watch. If she didn't do some of them, she either does them immediately, makes a note to carry those into the following week, or checks them off the list as no longer relevant. Keith does something similar, using the Full Focus Planner.

Every month, we try to get away on some kind of longer retreat, either for work or with friends or one of our tribes, or go to a conference, seminar, or training. Sometimes it's Burning Man, maybe it's a family reunion, but we rarely ever stay home for more than a month. We need to break that work cycle for our mental health. Leading up to Paleo f(x) usually involves longer workdays and less traveling, but when it's over, we always go somewhere to recover.

At the end of each year, we spend some time focusing on and writing down what we want to manifest in the new year. The next year, before setting new goals, we reassess how we did in meeting last year's goals. This keeps us moving forward and helps us understand what we did and didn't accomplish, and why.

Your Plan

You can organize your day, week, month, and year any way you choose, of course, but organizing is the part that can spur you to act and inspire you to keep going. Here are some suggested templates for planning and executing your basic training.

Primal Uprising Day Planner

You can plan your day around what you have to do and also what you have to do *for you*. See if you can work in something for each of the pillars throughout the day. Nothing has to be big or time-consuming. An extra vegetable serving here, a meditation moment there, deciding *not* to buy something tempting you don't need, giving someone a hug.

At the end of this list is an Uprising Act: one small thing you can do to further your freedom, or the freedom of others. This could be as simple as sharing a video about Big Ag, voting with your dollars to support a soul-preneur, or getting together with friends to talk about what leaders in your community to support.

	MORNING	AFTERNOON	EVENING	NOTES
Personal To-Do				
Work To-Do				
Physical Pillar				
Mental Pillar				
Emotional Pillar				
Spiritual Pillar				
Financial Pillar				

	MORNING	AFTERNOON	EVENING	NOTES
Relational Pillar				
Tribal Pillar				
Uprising Act				

Monthly Goals

See if you can find one big project you want to accomplish each month. These can be seasonal or organized in order of importance.

Month	Project
January	
February	
March	
April	
May	
June	
July	
August	
September	
October	
November	
December	

New Year's Day Plan

How did last year go, and what is your plan and intention for next year? Fill this out and keep it handy for reference all year long.

Last Year Analysis:
New Year Intentions:
Physical Pillar Goals:
Mental Pillar Goals:
Emotional Pillar Goals:

Spiritual Pillar Goals:

Financial Pillar Goals:

Relational Pillar Goals:

Tribal Pillar Goals:

Uprising Acts:

What do I want my life to look like one year from now?

20

THE WORLD BEYOND THE ZOO

Any jackass can kick down a barn, but it takes a carpenter to build one.

—Sam Rayburn

The final inspiration we want to give you is a glimpse of what the world could look like beyond the human zoo. At the beginning of this book, we took you through our view of the Bigs and what they have done to our world. In this chapter, we propose solutions and demonstrate how many of those solutions have already begun to happen at the grassroots level. We ask: How can this be better? We have ideas, and we hope this will spark more ideas in you because the more we all use our creativity and human ingenuity to rise up and take back our world for the betterment of humans, the easier freedom will come. Will it take a revolution? Maybe. Can it be a matter of a gradual installation of new and better systems? Maybe. Or, perhaps it will be a combination of both: some institutions may come tumbling down, while others can be refurbished.

We strongly believe that everyone has a talent (or more than one), and that playing to your strengths will help you discover where your place will be in this exciting new world. Maybe you're the activist type, or maybe you'd rather stay quietly in your home and plan, design, write, or meditate to raise the collective vibration. You do you—fully you, in optimal health, free from manipulation—and you will find your place in the new world.

What are your skills? What are your passions? What is your superpower? What gets you out of bed every morning? When you know what you want and what you love, you will be able to fit into the framework of the world you want to build.

If we want a better future, we need a better planet. If we want a better planet, we need better nations. If we want better nations, we need better cities. If we want better cities, we need better tribes. If we want better tribes, we need better people.

So let's build better people. Let's reverse-engineer this whole process from the future, all the way back to you. The primal uprising starts with you, as you re-envision your body, your health, your mind, your emotions, your spiritual life, your money, your relationships, your tribe, and the whole world. The more you grow personally, the better you will understand what your values are and the better you'll be able to live your truth and see the human zoo for what it is: an outmoded, corrupt, collapsing set of institutions that, unless we consent, don't have the power to hold us captive at all. This is the way to begin taking back our lives, our tribes, our nations, and our planet. This is how we build a future in which we can all be healthy, strong, clear-minded, and free.

As we go through each of the Bigs and what might (or already has begun to) replace them, listen for that still small voice inside of you whispering: *This! This is for me! This is where I can make a difference!* And then? Make a difference. We're right there with you.

Beyond Big Ag

Grassroots efforts are underway to restore the soil and incorporate agriculture into the ecosystem in a more sustainable way. We can do this, even make it profitable, but we have to be willing to move away from the old model. We believe the best way forward is to decentralize the agricultural system.

People often argue against an overhaul of the food system, saying that the more natural model isn't sustainable to feed our large population. This is simply not true. Remember the millions of buffaloes that used to roam our country from top to bottom? That was enough free-range meat to feed everyone. If we hadn't slaughtered most of them (often just for "sport") in a tragic mismanagement of natural resources, we could have lived in harmony with them—they could have continued to feed us, while we made sure they could continue to live their lives.

BRING BACK THE BISON (AND THE ELK AND THE DEER)

How many people can a bison feed? They are massive animals, and we've seen a butchery operation process a bison and get eight hundred pounds of meat. We were also able to witness that animal's humane harvesting. He was killed reverently. There was no panic, fear, or stress. He was dropped with one quick shot from a rifle at about seventy-five yards, and none of the other bison even looked up. They just kept eating. Bison have so much character. When we got to see them being moved from one paddock to another, they knew they were about to get fresh new grass so they were running and jumping, body-slamming each other and almost dancing for joy. Those bison had happy, natural lives.

One bison could feed a large family for a whole winter. There are other large game animals that could be similarly efficient sources for food, such as elk and deer. Millions of deer are "culled" every year where they have overpopulated. Why aren't we eating them? We kill deer, then buy cheap ground beef in the supermarket. There is no reason to waste the lives of those animals.

The reason the Midwest has had so much topsoil for so many centuries is because of the bison. Imagine hundreds of thousands of bison roaming the prairie, digging and scooping up the dirt with their hooves, fertilizing it with their dung, trimming the grass, then moving on to the next area. The wild birds come in after, pecking and scratching, fertilizing and seeding with the seeds in their droppings. The great thing is it doesn't take hundreds of years to regenerate topsoil this way. This has been proven by the

Savory Institute—they took a deforested, depleted ranch and put hoofed animals on it. They let them roam, and within twenty-four months, the soil had regenerated from desert to pastureland. There's no reason we can't do it all across the central US.

This is still possible on a more local scale. Any farmer can introduce hoofed animals to regenerate the topsoil that has virtually disappeared from the breadbasket of middle America.

You can watch how this works—*The Biggest Little Farm* is a great documentary about how a small family farm regenerated their soil with ingenuity and the help of animals. Joel Salatin, of Polyface Farm, is another example of the future of sustainable agriculture. Polyface runs on principles of sustainability, regeneration, soil health, and healthy, humanely treated livestock. It's the way people did things before the Bigs took over our food system and instituted monocropping/monoculture.

At Polyface Farm, animals live naturally and are harvested ethically. Joel and his crew rotate everything from paddock to parcel, moving the animals every six to eight hours, and they regularly shift where they grow each crop. This takes some doing at first, and a whole lot of microdecisions, but once the system is set up, it works fluidly and efficiently, and regenerates rather than depletes the soil.

Joel receives zero subsidies from the government, but guess what? His farm is actually incredibly profitable. You *can* make a living doing the right thing for your health and the environment, and you should be able to make a living doing something you feel makes a positive impact.

Imagine the Polyface Farm model popping up all over the country. Certain crops and livestock thrive in Joel's Virginia climate, but other farms in other parts of the country would produce different food. It would be in each farmer's best interest to grow the crops that did the best in that region. If all farms ran this way, we would all eat more seasonally. However, collaboration could result in the ability to get food from other parts of the country or the world (like avocados from California or seafood from Maine) . . . as long as you were willing to pay to have it shipped. For the least environmental impact and the freshest food, of course, it makes the most sense to eat primarily based on food that is locally produced and seasonal.

99 COUNTIES

Nick Wallace is a fourth-generation Iowa farmer who is assembling a collective of small family farms to provide food throughout the Midwest in exactly the kind of decentralized model we envision. These are his thoughts about the future of food:

I often daydream while I drive the back roads of Iowa. There isn't much to look at these days. Rows and rows of corn and soybeans, the occasional hog confinement, and abandoned farmhouses with crumbling barns. The small towns that dot the countryside have a faint pulse . . . maybe a convenience store and bar serving fried food with ranch dressing. The "Norman Rockwell" warm and fuzzy feeling of the past might be what the rest of the country envisions, but those days are but a distant memory.

Government policy during the last forty years has slowly turned a once self-sustainable and self-reliable farmer into an industrial tool of agribusiness. They don't have a choice to grow something besides corn and soybeans. But I see the potential for so much more. Emerald-green pastures dotted with cows, sheep, goats, chickens, turkeys, and ducks. A micro-dairy or two for each county, producing fresh raw milk, artisan cheese, cottage cheese, butter, and ice cream. The whey, a by-product, feeds the chickens for eggs. The eggs go to town with the neighbor's organic red winter wheat for the corner bakery. That bakery sells buns to the local burger joint. The burger joint uses the grass-fed local beef and the cheese from the dairy. Don't forget about the vegetable farmer who provides the lettuce, tomato, and pickles for the burger. Add some organic potatoes for the best French fries you've ever had. The burger joint buys lard from the acorn-and-apple-finished pork producer down the road. You haven't had French fries until you've had them fried in lard. The neighbor's hogs provide the meat for hot dogs, in case you're not in the mood for a burger. The orchard's best apples, peaches, blueberries, and strawberries go to the

> baker who makes pies, with crusts made of organic red
> winter wheat and lard. What if we could make this dream
> a reality?
>
> There are ninety-nine counties in Iowa, and 99 Counties
> is a venture that will become a vertically integrated, for-profit
> model for building health and vitality from the soil up. We
> have a network of farmers across the state ready and willing
> to farm thousands of acres regeneratively. A core of like-
> minded regenerative farmers have stepped forward, and we
> are building a better model, something larger than any one
> farmer could achieve alone. We have identified strengths and
> weaknesses throughout the "soil to plate" approach and are
> creating solutions to embolden farmers and consumers alike.
> Keep an eye out for us—we'll start in Iowa, but our goal is to
> provide real food for the entire US.

All the old arguments for supporting these industrial farming models are falling away, but people don't know what they don't know. You can spread the word, vote with your dollars for small family farms, buy grass-fed, pastured, wild-caught meat and seafood, diversify your diet, know the source of your food, tell your children, and let your friends know why you shop for food the way you do. Whether you buy from organic farmers through a CSA or stop at farm stands along the road or stock your freezer with meat from a local butcher, you will be making a difference, at the most basic level, and that difference will eventually trickle *up*.

Beyond Big Pharma and Big Medicine

To move beyond Big Pharma and Big Medical will require physical health, plain and simple. A strong, healthy, vital person will only occasionally need medical or pharmaceutical intervention, so prioritizing health is how we go beyond these Bigs. When these systems are no longer profitable, they might collapse—and we say *Good riddance!* In their place, we could have a decentralized model of medical care as we once did—small family practices that refer patients to specialists only when they genuinely need more advanced care.

If all we have are drugs and surgery, it's like trying to build a beautiful house with only a hammer. A hammer is a useful tool, but you can't build an entire house with it—you also need to be able to dig, sand, caulk, and so on, and those processes require other tools. For our bodies, the other tools we all have access to are nutrition, exercise, and stress management. We envision a future in which doctors teach us about prevention rather than spending most of their time trying to fix our problems.

When Michelle broke her ankle last year, we were grateful that she could go to a conventional doctor and have the broken bone set, but when she was offered surgery, she said no. She wanted to let her ankle heal naturally, and it healed just fine with time, care, and good nutrition. But hooray that we live in a time when orthopedic surgery is an option!

Option is the key. Drugs and surgery should be options, not requirements. Michelle wasn't going to visit a functional medicine doctor or get acupuncture for a broken bone, but for chronic conditions, we highly value our functional medicine and holistic doctors. We still need medical research, too. For example, bacteria are good at mutating to outsmart the antibiotics we have, so we need to keep developing antibiotics that can save the lives of those who get infections from resistant bacteria. If one of us were to get sepsis from an antibiotic-resistant bacteria, we're going to hope and pray that a pharmaceutical solution exists.

When we are all healthier, we may discover that those who do develop diseases are those with genetic propensities, so knowing your genetics can give you a leg up on those genetic risk factors. This is becoming increasingly easy—there are many companies offering genetic tests that can let you know where you might be susceptible. Genetic testing can also tell you what medication might or might not work for you. If you are susceptible to heart disease, diabetes, autoimmunity, or cancer, you can use that valuable information as motivation to stay as healthy as possible. Do this in your teens or early twenties, and get your baseline biomarkers so you know what's normal for you, and you will be significantly empowered to manage your own health and monitor any changes from your own healthy normal.

We also believe it's best to focus on integrative medicine as a legitimate form of care. Functional, integrative, alternative, naturopathic, and osteopathic doctors are focused on why you have healthcare problems, and addressing the root causes of those problems, rather than covering up your symptoms with drugs. Because many of them don't take insurance (because insurance companies refuse to cover their services), they may cost more up front, but when it comes to managing wellness and addressing chronic issues, there is no better way to get the thorough attention you need from someone who will look at you in the context of your entire life, not just your headache or your sore knee. In the long run, you are likely to save money because you will get the tools to become healthy, rather than having to keep going back into the system.

But before someone needs to go to a doctor, they could, in a future world, be armed with the knowledge to stay healthy in the first place. We believe the healthcare system of the future will be grounded in nutritional counseling, physical training, and mental health maintenance. We can imagine that the first-line healthcare model will start in the gym.

Picture a full-service gym with trainers, nutritionists, health coaches, and counselors. There could be swimming pools, running tracks, saunas, and massage therapists. Health coaches could help people optimize the seven pillars. What if everybody did that first? We'd have a lot fewer sick people to start with, but when people do need doctors, we can envision a system based on concierge doctors. You pay your personal doctor for what you need, and get tax incentives to finance healthcare when you need it. Health insurance could be woven into this system based on a more personalized medicine model, and concierge doctors could guide not only prevention but human optimization. This would mean, of course, that medical schools would also transition to a curriculum that included detailed and rigorous training on prevention and optimization.

Why wait? There are already health coaches all over the country. Vote with your dollars for preventive care and choose not to engage with Big Pharma and Big Medical unless you absolutely have to.

REED DAVIS SAYS . . .

Is evidence-based medicine (EBM) the "gold standard" in medical care? Not quite, says Reed Davis, Founder of Functional Diagnostic Nutrition:

> What's missing in the EBM model is an individualized investigation into why a person has medical issues in the first place. Not just a quick diagnosis and treatment or management of disease approach, but a deep dive into the underlying causes found upstream in the complexities of one's metabolism.

Beyond Big Business

Money is energy, and energy can be fuel for innovation. When we look to the future, we see Big Business as decentralized, just like Big Ag. We envision a much more vigorous gig economy with entrepreneurs creating innovations based on the seven pillars. We envision widespread abundance and an economy based on people first, with profit following because of that life-centered, health-centered, mission-centered focus.

Money, as we've already established, is not good or bad, but the more money you make, the more energy you have for innovation, and that is what drives this movement forward. You can use your money to buy your next yacht or your next Learjet, but people in this community are realizing that money can be used for something better than that. There is so much more beyond personal gain. Money gives you the freedom to ask: What can I create next? What can I do in collaboration with others? It's an abundance mindset rather than a scarcity mindset.

So, what do Airbnb, Uber, Bitcoin, Waze, and MakeSoil have in common (just to name a few)? They are all examples of decentralized, crowd-sourced businesses succeeding despite the odds in an environment that favors centralized corporate structures. What will save us all are the entrepreneurs who can build the new systems. One of our commitments is to support new entrepreneurs who are passionate about their causes but are just learning how to be businesspeople. Whether they are developing technologies to overhaul global transportation or they make cookies with wholesome ingredients, they can be part of the new economy. Can a cookie change the world? Sure it can, when it changes perspective and shows you that you have options.

We've noticed something interesting about the younger generation in the workforce—they are less interested in profit and that old concept of the American dream (big house, fancy car, retirement plan) and more interested in flexibility, passion, life experience, and freedom. They reject the idea of being tied down by debt, mortgages, or even cars. When an entire generation comes up fast knowing exactly what they want, and when what they want isn't material, it could transform the entire model. We are steadily moving away from the cubicle and into the home office, despite what Big Business might like to see. There is a sea change happening out there, driven by entrepreneurs—we believe that in the new economy, everyone is an entrepreneur, or at least, has the mindset of one. Invest in yourself and you'll discover a whole new set of priorities for your money and time (we recommend reading *The Last Safe Investment*, by Bryan Franklin and Michael Ellsberg).

There are thousands of examples of genius soulpreneurs who are changing the world because they can, and because they want to make the world better. If that's also profitable, then good for them! That's just more energy to keep improving life for us all. We think Paleo f(x) itself is a model for a future economy that is freer and more ethical than the supposedly free market we have now. You can vote with your dollars to support businesses like these, rather than corporate giants who operate solely for profit.

JOSH WHITON SAYS . . .

Our friend Josh Whiton could retire ten times over but keeps innovating. He's an inventor who cofounded one of the first urban farms in the southern United States, integrated into Research Triangle Park in North Carolina. Most recently, he founded MakeSoil.org, which registers public and private compost bins. He points out that the health of the soil is critical to the health of the whole planet, and has made a successful business out of this very important mission:

> Nearly everyone is contributing in some way to the decline of Earth's soil. But what if nearly everyone could contribute to restoring it? We can't expect the soil to produce quality food for us endlessly unless we give back to that soil. How? Through the miracle of composting. You can think of composting as a recipe. It means mixing nitrogen-rich food scraps together with carbon-rich things like dry grass, sawdust, or leaves, adding the right amount of moisture, the right amount of airflow, and *kaboom*—a whole microbial world will wake up, get busy, get hot, and go about turning all those food scraps into new, living, soil. A handful of living soil is like a little galaxy, a microcosm, containing countless life forms, in countless numbers. Such soil is an ecosystem unto itself. If all life on Earth were to be extinguished, but a handful of living soil survive, we might fast forward a billion or two years ahead and find advanced life-forms and civilization had once again emerged. Living soil can be part of a functional ecosystem in a way that dead dirt can't. Living soil not only makes for stronger, healthier plants, but it can keep the rest of nature in balance too, helping to protect crops from blights and other catastrophes that signal a lack of biodiversity and an ecosystem out of balance.

Where would you fit into this model? Ask yourself what your gifts are. In the world beyond the zoo, everyone will be able to work according to their own talents and passions. How could you contribute to a more decentralized economy? Are you creative? Good at science? An engineering genius? Are you a builder, planner, manifester, healer, maker? Do you have ideas for the environment, clean energy, a new food system? Do you have an idea we haven't begun to think of?

Who says you can't change the world with your idea? The more people who get out there and try, the less reliant we will be on a consumerist economy that keeps us chained to a life that is only about making money to buy more stuff, and the bigger we can grow an economy that frees us to live according to our values.

We believe that decentralization is the *only* answer. We need to buy locally, just like with our food. We need to be willing to pay a little more on the front end, as an investment in our own economies, and most importantly, we need to take back control of our attention. Let's look up from the screens and the social media feeds and the addictive ads and videos that shape our thoughts, and try thinking for ourselves again, so we can reclaim our creativity and reinvent what it means to work.

Beyond Big Government and Big Military

It's probably no big secret that we lean Libertarian, and that may be why we see a future where government is largely decentralized and should never be able to overrule or override state and local governments. We still need a federal government to defend us when necessary (which should be the one and only job of the military, free from profit motive and corporate influence), make sure our civil liberties aren't violated, intercede in disaster scenarios, and manage infrastructure. We need them for interstate highways and air traffic control, and a few other important, key jobs, but that's it. They have way too much power and way too much control over state and local governments who know their people better.

We think this will begin with the dismantling of the two-party system. It's already happening at the local level. Every so often, someone runs on an independent ticket, and sometimes they even win. This is where we need to put our efforts—not necessarily toward any one of those parties, but toward a system that disrupts the "either/or" mentality. Maybe the solution is many parties. Maybe the solution is no parties. Whatever it is, we need to change what we have now if we ever hope to have a country led by those who actually care about and vote according to the needs of the citizenry.

One powerful way to make that change would be to institute term limits. We believe there should be no career politicians. Right now, there are politicians in government at the national level, on both sides, who have been there for thirty, forty, fifty years. Their argument is that they have experience, but what have we gotten for all of this experience? When they say, "We know how the system works," what we hear is, "We know how the wheel gets greased. We know how to line our pockets." Many of the so-called public servants running our government have become multimillionaires while serving in government. How did we let that happen? Serving in government is supposed to be about serving, not getting rich. As soon as there is profit potential, we can almost guarantee there will be corruption.

The original purpose of representatives was that the elected officials would do their civic duty by serving their communities, states, or country, and then when their terms were over, they would go home and get back to their businesses or whatever they were doing before. If you get perks because you are in business, fine, but when you are a lawmaker, you shouldn't be getting perks, kickbacks, and blatant payoffs from lobbyists to influence your vote. Of course that can become so irresistible that you never want to go back to your other life. The temptation to use an elected position to line one's own pockets or blackmail other lawmakers into voting a certain way is large and real. If we continue to allow people to be career politicians, we are going to keep getting what we've got.

If we want change, we have to vote them out. Every single one of them. That's the only way we're ever going to get out of systemic corruption. Just look at the world—financial collapse, rogue nations running around with nuclear weapons, corporations considered to be humans, countries vying for power and financial leverage, and a government that tells us what we can and can't do at every level. Vote them out: this is how we avoid another housing crisis, another financial crisis, another scandal. Let's wipe the slate clean!

Beyond Big Banking

It's hard to imagine taking down Big Banking because of its secretive nature and covert operation, with its tentacles in all the other Bigs, but it all begins with each one of us getting out from under their thumb: out of debt and the consumerist, materialistic mindset that got us there. Meanwhile, will we accept "Too big to fail" from them ever again, or are we going to demand they pay for what they have done to our economy time and time again?

A disruption of one of those big entities would likely be a legitimate major financial blow to the economy, but that may be just the reset we need to finally decentralize the banks. If we don't, it's going to keep happening. Vote with your attention so the career politicians who were all involved in giving the thumbs-up to that bail-out, who all made money off the American people, never get the chance to commit fraud on the American people again.

This will require a complete change in priorities for many people. It may take a while, but it could be a reality if we all decide to make it work. This is a job for a tribe because nobody is an island, and survival is (as it always has been) a team sport. We're working on this for ourselves right now, planning how to live off the grid, but there are many ways to free yourself from Big Banking. When we all support each other with our talents and skills, we can live in a world beyond financial control.

Wealth doesn't have to be money. It can be (and was for most of human history) about resources, and resources can be shared, traded, and maximized for the greater good. For us, that looks like a community where everyone works together, growing vegetables, raising chickens and goats, tending Jersey cows that produce milk, making cheese, building houses, sewing clothes, hunting and cooking food, hooking up solar panels, building generators, teaching children, writing books—if this rustic kind of scenario doesn't appeal to you, don't let that limit you. It sounds like utopia to us, but there are many ways local communities could look in a world where the Bigs have no sway. Let your imagination run away with you. Imagine what your ideal life would be like. Picture a society based on human worth rather than money. Find those who share your vision, and start building. What's stopping you?

Escaping Big Banking is about more than resources. It's also about sanity, human interaction, love, and the prioritization of the real rather than the fake. It's human life driven by what is best in humanity, rather than what is worst. It is to live the way we were always meant to live.

. . .

There is a world beyond the Bigs and we think it's coming, like it or not. We can't tell you exactly what it will look like, but it seems to us there are two options: The End, or The Beginning.

Let's be ready to replace what comes down with something better. Rather than wandering through the ashes of a world gone wrong, we can become the architects of the future, each and every one of us. Every human being has the capacity to contribute positively to the entire planet, and if we all chose to do that—wow! When we all work together, we can do anything.

We have the potential to become an integrated and vigorously evolving planet full of optimally healthy world citizens working together to recapture what we have lost and carry it proudly into the future. This is what will save humanity from itself, so let's make it happen. Let's all decide to be better people than we are today. Now you have the playbook. You know what you need to do. Let's do it together, in unity. Let's rise.

Acknowledgments

So many people over the years have contributed to the knowledge that has resulted in this book. We can't possibly thank them all individually. There are some who have been particularly and more directly influential, whom we do want to mention. This book would not have been possible without the encouragement and support of Jaidree Braddix at Park & Fine and the excellent team at BenBella: Glenn Yeffeth, Claire Schulz, Karen Wise, Jessika Rieck, Sarah Avinger, Heather Butterfield, Kim Broderick, Greg Teague, and Jennifer Canzoneri. Thanks also to Eve Adamson, for being such an integral and important partner in the creation of this book. We couldn't have written the book we ended up with, without your guidance and expertise. Without you involved, this book would've been good—however, thankfully, with you involved, it's *excellent*! You were able to marry our individual voices, thoughts, and ideas in a way we never could have. We love you; you're family.

We'd also like to thank the many people who took the time to contribute their thoughts and ideas and who are quoted directly or indirectly in this book, including Robb Wolf, Dave Asprey, Tah Whitty, Brandon Yager, Dr. Lisa Whitty Bradley, Theo Wilson, Dr. Mickra Hamilton, Darryl Edwards, Ben Greenfield, Dr. Guillermo Ruiz, Reed Davis, Shawn Wells, Krisstina Wise, Jolie Dawn, Abel James, Barbara Ditlow, Hal Elrod, Molly Maloof, Kyle Kingsbury, Pete Evans, Erwan Le Corre, Abbie Sawyer, Dr. Chris LoRang, Dr. Andy Galpin, Charlie Deist, David Nurse,

Mark England, David Berceli, Paul Chek, Logan Stout, Nick Wallace, Josh Whiton, Luis Villaseñor, and Dr. Christopher Ryan.

Paleo f(x) was of course the genesis for this book, so we would be remiss if we didn't include the key people involved in the evolution of Paleo f(x). Instrumental in the birth of Paleo f(x): Shirley McLean, Erik Schimek, and Alex Baia. Thanks also to our current *rockstar* Paleo f(x) team: Jia Raneses-Lao, Janet Joy Rubrico, Christian Rea, Lauren Pena, John Marc Adalid, Angel Faith Bernaldo, Chase Panozzo, Rahul Sangave, and Celia Grace Garcia Guerrero, and to former team members Melissa Wilbert, Misty Williams, Danielle Gordon, Diana Lane, Peter Bauman, Sara Gustafson, Kristen Waltrip, Kiersten Peterson, Benjamin Nutt, Alex Baia, Lauren Maxwell, Kimberly Pope, Frances Smith, Steven Reinoehl, Clayton Miller, Christal McMillion, Cassi McHenry, Nick VerDuin, Anna Dooley, and Jayci Cormier. Your contributions were invaluable to the growth of Paleo f(x). For being our speaker coordinator since year one we must thank Rachel Flowers. We owe her so much! Thanks also to all our speakers, sponsors, exhibitors, and attendees, both past and present, who have been and remain an essential and integral part of our Paleo f(x) family. Please know that if you are a part of our movement, you have our deepest thanks for the support. And to the people who were not just huge supporters of Paleo f(x) but have also supported us personally through everything, you can't know how much it means to us for you to stand by us in the way you have: Frank Priebe, Leanna Cappucci, Todd McVay, Susan Maupin, Jules Chavez, Debbie Torrance, and Robin Eacret.

We also need to thank our families, including Keith's parents, Carl and Nancy Norris; Michelle's mom, Judi Mull; Michelle's niece, Morgan Dear, and Michelle's aunt, Jacque Kahre.

And speaking of families, for personal, spiritual, and professional support, we have relied deeply on our SoulFam: Rick Hamilton, Tah and Kole Whitty, Dr. Dan Stickler, Dr. Mickra Hamilton, Brandon and Deb Yager, Barbara Ditlow, Jennifer Goodman, Dr. Elena Villanueva, Greg Platz, Boris Peysakhov, Krisstina Wise, Shawn Wells, Clayton Miller, Giselle Koy, Kristina Ensminger, Stephanie Bellinger, Heather Havenwood, Ron

Michael, Lee Noto, Ani Manian, Michelle Alderman, Dr. Kaylea Bednarz Boutwell, JR Burgess, Kayla Osterhoff, Kristi Holt, Dr. Torrie Thompson, Amy Wharton, Jess Poitra, Zach Poitra, John Cole, and especially J. J. Virgin, without whom this book might never have come to fruition. JJ not only introduced us to our agent, she was the biggest supporter of this book and she endorsed us with such confidence that she convinced Michelle we could write it. JJ, you'll never know how much that meant to us.

Thank you for every time you were there for us when we needed you: Shannan Canavan Ford, Jennifer Moran, Betty Jean Bell, David Gonzalez, Wendy Ryan, and Mike Dillard. We also could not do without the love, support, and adventures with our Burning Man family, Soulpreneur f(x) family, RP Badasses Group, our IDLifeWellness family, and Michelle's Rebel Road Sistas led by her partner in crime, Jennifer Moran. You all know who you are and we love you more than we could ever express in words.

Last but certainly not least, on the most personal of notes, we thank our children: our daughters, Brittani Panozzo and Kaley Norris; our sons, Chase Panozzo and Kleat Norris; and our grandson, Dominick Oltmanns; thank you all for continuing to inspire us to want to create a better world. We love you more than words can ever express.

We must also say that we deeply and passionately thank each other, because none of this would have happened if we had not found each other again and combined our energies with love, hope, and purpose.

Notes

1. Shahla Hosseini Bai and Steven M. Ogbourne, "Glyphosate: Environmental Contamination, Toxicity and Potential Risks to Human Health via Food Contamination," *Environmental Science and Pollution Research* 23 (2016): 18988–9001, doi.org/10.1007/s11356-016-7425-3.

2. Institutes of Medicine (US) Committee to Review the Health Effects in Vietnam Veterans of Exposure to Herbicides, *Veterans and Agent Orange: Health Effects of Herbicides Used in Vietnam* (Washington, DC: National Academies Press, 1994), ncbi.nlm.nih.gov/books/NBK236351.

3. Melissa Denchak, "Flint Water Crisis: Everything You Need to Know," Natural Resources Defense Council, November 8, 2018, www.nrdc.org/stories/flint-water-crisis-everything-you-need-know.

4. Joe Neel, "Medical Schools and Drug Firm Dollars," NPR, June 9, 2005, www.npr.org/templates/story/story.php?storyId=4696316.

5. James Hamblin, "Why the Government Pays Billions to People Who Claim Injury by Vaccines," *The Atlantic*, May 14, 2019, theatlantic.com/health/archive/2019/05/vaccine-safety-program/589354.

6. Nolan Feeney, "Pentagon: 7 in 10 Youths Would Fail to Qualify for Military Service," *Time*, June 29, 2014, time.com/2938158/youth-fail-to-qualify-military-service.

7. Moody's Analytics, "The Economic Consequences of Millennial Health," Blue Cross Blue Shield, November 6, 2019, bcbs.com/the-health-of-america/reports/how-millennials-current-and-future-health-could-affect-our-economy.

8. For an interesting look at the problems with our election system and how we might fix it, see Jameson Quinn, "'Ranked Choice Voting'? I Support It, but . . .": May 16, 2018, medium.com/@jameson.quinn/ranked-choice-voting-i-support-it-but-679e96b1b5f0.

9. For a simple introduction to how this works, watch Clayton Traylor's You-Tube video "SIMPLE Easy to Understand 3-Minute Video on the Federal Reserve" (youtu.be/njFrqTJx0mI). Traylor also has an interesting book—from a religious perspective, FYI—on this subject and more. It's just one person's point of view, but it could be a jumping-off point for more research, if you are so inclined.

10. Bruce K. Alexander, "Addiction: The View from Rat Park," brucekalexander.com, 2010, brucekalexander.com/articles-speeches/rat-park/148-addiction-the-view-from-rat-park.

11. Herman Pontzer, Brian M. Wood, and David A. Raichlen, "Hunter-Gatherers as Models in Public Health," *Obesity Reviews*, December 3, 2018, doi/full.org/10.1111/obr.12785.

12. Monica Barone et al., "Gut Microbiome Response to a Modern Paleolithic Diet in a Western Lifestyle Context," PLoS One 14, no. 8 (August 8, 2019): e0220619, doi.org/10.1371/journal.pone.0220619.

13. Rachel Rettner, "One Company's Hand Sanitizer Products Contain Potentially Deadly Substance, FDA Warns," LiveScience.com, June 23, 2020, livescience.com/hand-sanitizer-methanol-fda-warning.html.

14. Bill Hesselmar et al., "Pet-Keeping in Early Life Reduces the Risk of Allergy in a Dose-Dependent Fashion," *PLoS One*, December 19, 2018, doi.org/10.1371/journal.pone.0208472.

15. National Center for Advancing Translational Sciences, "Understanding the Brain's Response to Sugar Could Help Treat Obesity," National Institutes of Health, updated October 26, 2018, ncats.nih.gov/pubs/features/understanding-brains-response; Eleanor Busby et al., "Mood Disorders and Gluten: It's Not All in Your Mind! A Systematic Review of Meta-Analysis," *Nutrients* 10, no. 11 (November 2018), doi.org/10.3390/nu10111708.

16. Magalie Lenoir et al., "Intense Sweetness Surpasses Cocaine Reward," *PLoS One* 2, no. 8 (August 1, 2007): e698, doi.org/10.1371/journal.pone.0000698.

17. Paola Bressan and Peter Kramer, "Bread and Other Edible Agents of Mental Disease," *Frontiers in Human Neuroscience* 10 (March 29, 2016), doi.org/10.3389/fnhum.2016.00130.

18. Andy R. Eugene and Jolanta Masiak, "The Neuroprotective Aspects of Sleep," MEDtube Sci 3, no. 1 (March 2015): 35–40, medtube.net/science/wp-content/uploads/2014/03/The-Neuroprotective-Aspects-of-Sleep.pdf.

19. Simon Makin, "Deep Sleep Gives Your Brain a Deep Clean," *Scientific American*, November 1, 2019, scientificamerican.com/article/deep-sleep-gives-your-brain-a-deep-clean1.

20. Benson M. Hoffman et al., "Exercise and Pharmacotherapy in Patients with Major Depression: One-Year Follow-Up of the SMILE Study," *Psychosomatic Medicine* 73, no. 2 (February–March 2011): 127–133, doi.org/10.1097/PSY .0b013e31820433a5.

21. American Academy of Pediatrics, "Combining Physical Activity with Classroom Lessons Results in Improved Test Scores," ScienceDaily, July 1, 2011, sciencedaily.com/releases/2011/05/110501183653.htm.

22. Sammi R. Chekroud et al., "Association Between Physical Exercise and Mental Health in 1.2 Million Individuals in the USA Between 2011 and 2015: A Cross-Sectional Study," *The Lancet Psychiatry* 5, no. 9 (September 1, 2018): 739–46, doi.org/10.1016/S2215-0366(18)30227-X.

23. Gregory N. Bratman et al., "Nature and Mental Health: An Ecosystem Service Perspective," *Science Advances* 5, no. 7 (July 24, 2019), doi.org/10.1126/sciadv .aax0903.

24. Sue Penckofer et al., "Vitamin D and Depression: Where Is All the Sunshine?" *Issues in Mental Health Nursing* 31, no. 6 (June 2010): 385–393, doi.org/10 .3109/01612840903437657.

25. National Center for Complementary and Integrative Health, "Meditation: In Depth," National Institutes of Health, updated April 2016, nccih.nih.gov /health/meditation-in-depth.

26. Menelaos L. Batrinos, "Testosterone and Aggressive Behavior in Men," *International Journal of Endocrinology and Metabolism* 10, no. 3 (Summer 2012): 563–68, doi.org/10.5812/ijem.3661; Bronwyn M. Graham et al., "Sex Hormones Are Associated with Rumination and Interact with Emotion Regulation Strategy Choice to Predict Negative Affect in Women Following a Sad Mood Induction," *Frontiers in Psychology* 9 (2018): 937, doi.org/10.3389/fpsyg.2018.00937.

27. Linda Owen, "Distorting the Past. Gender and the Division of Labor in the European Upper Paleolithic," *PaleoAnthropology* (2008): 91–92, paleoanthro .org/static/journal/content/PA20080091.pdf.

28. M. Dyble et al., "Sex Equality Can Explain the Unique Structure of Hunter-Gatherer Bands," *Science* 348, no. 6236 (May 15, 2015): 796–98, doi.org/10 .1126/science.aaa5139.

29. Rollin McCraty, Raymond Trevor Bradley, and Dana Tomasino, "The Resonant Heart," *Shift: At the Frontiers of Consciousness,* December 2004–February 2005, heartmath.org/assets/uploads/2015/01/the-resonant-heart.pdf.

30. Harold G. Koenig, "Religion, Spirituality, and Health: The Research and Clinical Implications," *ISRN Psychiatry* 2012 (December 16, 2012), doi.org/10 .5402/2012/278730.

31. "Help Others," Mental Health America, accessed October 23, 2020, mhanational.org/help-others.

32. Michael Lipka and Claire Gecewicz, "More Americans Now Say They're Spiritual but Not Religious," Pew Research Center, September 6, 2017, pewresearch.org/fact-tank/2017/09/06/more-americans-now-say-theyre -spiritual-but-not-religious.

33. Sherrie Hurd, "What Is Schumann Resonance and How It Is Connected to Human Consciousness," Learning-Mind.com, June 30, 2019, learning-mind .com/schumann-resonance-human-consciousness.

34. Foundation for Shamanic Studies, "The Way of the Shaman: The Work of Michael and Sandra Harner," Shamanism.org, accessed November 6, 2020, shamanism.org/way-of-the-shaman/documentary.php;scienceandnondu- ality, "The Transcendence of Time in Shamanic Practice, Michael Harner, SAND 2011," YouTube, accessed December 9, 2020, youtu.be/27DCN0f_1fc.

35. Nathan Bomey and John Gallagher, "How Detroit Went Broke: The Answers May Surprise You—and Don't Blame Coleman Young," *Detroit Free Press,* July 18, 2018, freep.com/story/news/local/michigan/detroit/2013/09/15/how -detroit-went-broke-the-answers-may-surprise-you-and/77152028.

36. Daniel Kahneman and Angus Deaton, "High Income Improves Evaluation of Life but Not Emotional Well-Being," *PNAS* 107, no. 38 (September 21, 2010): 16489–93, doi.org/10.1073/pnas.1011492107.

37. Robert Frank, "The Perfect Income for Happiness? It's $161,000," CNBC, November 30, 2012, cnbc.com/id/50027184.

38. Norman Vanamee, "Here's Exactly How Much Money You Need to Be Happy," *Town & Country,* November 16, 2017, townandcountrymag.com/society/money -and-power/a13528013/how-much-money-you-need-to-be-happy.

39. "User Clip: Bush Shopping Quote," C-SPAN, October, 2011, c-span.org/video /?c4552776/user-clip-bush-shopping-quote.

40. Joshua Fields Millburn and Ryan Nicodemus, "What Is Minimalism?" The Minimalists, accessed October 28, 2020, theminimalists.com/minimalism.

41. Jennifer Calonia, "Average American Debt," Bankrate, March 23, 2020, bankrate.com/finance/debt/average-american-debt.

42. Jessica Martino, Jennifer Pegg, and Elizabeth Pegg Frates, "The Connection Prescription: Using the Power of Social Interactions and the Deep Desire for Connectedness to Empower Health and Wellness," *American Journal of Life- style Medicine* 11, no. 6 (November–December 2017): 466–75, doi.org/10 .1177/1559827615608788.

43. Kevin deLaplante, "Within Polarized Tribes, Complexity is Unstable," You-Tube, October 31, 2020, youtu.be/PwGZrW5K97k; "In Our Tribe We Trust," YouTube, April 27, 2018, youtu.be/QjRf8C8XmFs; "Our Tribal Intelligence," YouTube, February 17, 2018, youtu.be/f3ZRFemh_7M; "The Dangers of Tribalism," YouTube, January 19, 2018, youtu.be/7y-b7f6CK2M.

44. Judith M. Burkart, Rahel K. Brügger, and Carel P. van Schaik, "Evolutionary Origins of Morality: Insights from Nonhuman Primates," *Frontiers in Sociology*, July 9, 2018, doi.org/10.3389/fsoc.2018.00017; Adina L. Roskies, "The Origins of Morality," *Nature* 472 (April 14, 2011), nature.com/articles/472166a.pdf.

Index

About the Authors

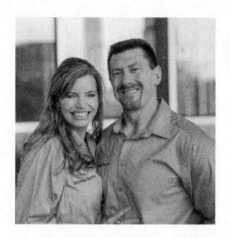

Michelle and Keith Norris are the cofounders of Paleo f(x)™, the largest-of-its-kind health and wellness platform and event in the world. They are passionate speakers and motivators to those seeking deliverance from a broken healthcare system and disabled economic system. Having left the corporate grind far behind, they are now serial entrepreneurs in the health and wellness space, as well as tireless firebrands for advancing the Paleo movement—a cultural reawakening of self-empowerment for the twenty-first century. In addition to leading the Paleo f(x) movement, Michelle and Keith speak at events and conferences worldwide on the topic of self-empowerment and breaking free of the human zoo.